BODY WISDOM

The wisdom lies within

J. Harper

To my parents and Celia Critchley
with much love

Body Wisdom

SELF-HEALING USING CHINESE AND
NATURAL MEDICINE

Jennifer Harper

Thorsons
An Imprint of HarperCollins*Publishers*

The Author

Jennifer Harper is a successful Natural Health Practitioner who is qualified and registered in a variety of holistic therapies. She is a gifted healer and runs her own clinic where she believes in treating the 'whole' person by using a combination of techniques including nutrition, Western and Chinese herbs, acupressure, reflexology, essential oils and flower remedies. Over many years, hundreds of people have been healed by Jennifer and guided towards a greater understanding of their body and health. Jennifer is also an accomplished and motivational broadcaster on television and radio.

Jennifer Harper can be contacted by writing the address below, enclosing a SAE:

PO Box 150
Woking
Surrey
GU23 6XS

Acknowledgements

I would like to thank my friends and colleagues for their love and support throughout the writing of *Body Wisdom*. My thanks to the following practitioners for their advice and verification of the content of the book: Dr Michael Tierra, Efrem Korngold, Jan de Vries, Edward Thompson, Andrew Sordyl, Jacqueline Young and Ruth Copland for her assistance with proofreading. A special thanks goes to Pierre Cousin for generously giving up his valuable time to scrutinize the text and provide information and artwork on the five elements for inclusion in the book. Thanks to agents Lisa Eveleigh and Jonathan Lloyd; and to my first editor, Jane Graham-Maw, for recognising my potential and encouraging me finally to write the book after carrying the idea around in my head for many years and to her successor, Wanda Whiteley, who has maintained the same level of encouragement. I would like to give John Clifford a special mention for all the support he has given me. Finally, thank you to all my patients who continue to reinforce my belief in the power of natural healing.

Whilst the author and the publishers have taken every care to check the text for accuracy, we cannot accept responsibility for any harm caused following the advice in this book. If you are suffering from any illness, always consult your doctor before following advice contained in this book.

Thorsons
An Imprint of HarperCollins*Publishers*
77–85 Fulham Palace Road,
Hammersmith, London W6 8JB
1160 Battery Street,
San Francisco, California 94111-1213
Published by Thorsons 1997

10 9 8 7 6 5 4 3 2

A catalogue record for this book
is available from the British Library

The diagrams on pages 5 and 7 are based on originals by Pierre J. Cousin.

ISBN 0 7225 3368 3

Printed and bound in Great Britain by
Creative Print and Design (Wales), Ebbw Vale

Contents

Foreword

It is with the greatest pleasure that I write the foreword for a book which is not only very impressive but looks at health in general from a completely different angle to that of most health books. The writer has gone into deep research of different alternative methods of how one can help oneself to better health. Along with the possible conventional approaches, there is a lot that patients can do to help their own doctors, consultants and therapists to improve their health mentally, physically and emotionally. Complementary medicine is looking at man not having one body but three: unless there is harmony in the physical, mental and emotional bodies, there will always be trouble. This book shows ways to look at these three bodies as, in today's society, we often see more problems of the third body, the emotional body, which is very often neglected and also a mighty weapon in one's own hands if one knows the ways to approach it. Whatever treatments, alternative or conventional, there is no improvement unless one has a positive mind. Positive action, in whatever treatment, will be of utmost importance as there is no improvement in health unless patients are relaxed and in full harmony with themselves and the people treating them. It needs a lot of self-education to arrive at this point.

I have known Jenni for many years and, when she was still quite young I was surprised at the terrific hunger and thirst that she had to help others. She studied, kept asking and asking and, in so doing, became a very busy student, educating herself and looking at all kinds of methods of helping others. It is this sharing which is so important in life; Jenni tries not only in her writing and in her personal consultations but also in her radio and television interviews to share with others what she has learned, and also the methods which she has tried which have worked and helped patients.

Today Jenni is trying to build bridges between orthodox medicine and alternative medicine to arrive at a complementary system which will help human suffering in more efficient ways. Orthodox medicine is a result of the technical revolution and has not been with us for very long. Alternative medicine has been with us for as long as we can remember and is defined as the original medicine. With all aspects of the two systems, which I have been practising for over 35 years, I have come to the conclusion that while a very sophisticated medicine can be of help, a very simple, long-forgotten herb can sometimes do the job even better. It is wonderful to see that, in today's society, these systems are coming more and more together, not only because of the changes in medicine which have taken place but because people like Jenni have put all their efforts into making the systems known and giving people freedom of choice in the way they are treated.

This is where a book like Jenni's fills a gap. It combines alternative treatments with other methods which have been proven to be successful. It is important that not just the obvious symptoms are cured, as conventional medicine teaches us. We have to look for the cause of the illness and, in looking at the cause, we come to understand how much we can do ourselves, with diet and simple methods which can be applied when necessary.

We learn every day that we have lost contact with grassroot levels. We have to realize that we belong to nature, we have to obey the laws of nature and, in so doing, we obey the laws of our creator. I am quite sure that this book will be of great help to many and, as Jenni has put so much effort into this, it will also be an eye-opener on long-proven methods which will improve your health and happiness.

Jan de Vries
D. Ho. Med., D.O., M.R.O., H.D., M.R.N., D.Ac, M.B.Ac

Introduction

While putting the finishing touches to *Body Wisdom*, I met a cardiac surgeon from Vienna, Dr Kassal Hermann. We were discussing the importance of health and how it is so often neglected or taken for granted. He told me a wonderful Austrian quote, which translates as:

> *Health is not everything, but without health everything is nothing.*

How many of us can say that we respect our bodies and value our health? Hippocrates, the Father of Medicine, appreciated the significance of good health when he said those famous words

> *A wise man ought to realize that health is his most valuable possession.*

Stress and strain seem to go hand in hand with life in the 20th century. More than ever before, we need to search for ways to re-establish harmony and equilibrium in our mind, body and spirit; to find a better way of taking care of ourselves by listening to our bodies and becoming more in tune with them. Do we know what our body is trying to tell us with the symptoms that it is displaying? These symptoms are so important as they are early warning signs that nature shows us in the hope that we can take preventative measures. The wise soul takes heed of these and will try to find the cause of the problem, as this is where the solution will be found and where self-healing begins.

In *Body Wisdom*, I outline my own unique holistic approach which greatly assists the process of self-healing. The main theme of the book focuses on the internal organs and their function in Western terms and the interpretation and significance of each organ according to Traditional Chinese Medicine (TCM). It is my desire to share with you this empowering knowledge about the importance of the inner organs of the body and what they can reveal, so that you will have a greater understanding of the wisdom that lies within.

When we seek to restore or build our levels of health, we gain the greatest results when working with a variety of healing methods which help to nourish and support weak organs and body systems. This book, therefore, includes a variety of 'holistic' methods (i.e. ones that balance the psychological, physical and spiritual levels) to help strengthen and create balance in the body. These methods acknowledge that the mind, body and spirit need to be treated as a living unity and are based on the fundamental belief that the individual plays a vital role in his or her own healing. The therapies are simple and highly effective and when combined with the wisdom of Chinese medicine, create an exciting new way of working with the body.

Incorporating the self-help measures outlined in this book can help you correct imbalances in their early stages – that is, before they develop into common illnesses.

> *A doctor who treats a disease after it has happened is a mediocre doctor ... a doctor who treats a disease before it happens is a superior doctor.*
> *Yellow Emperor's Classic of Internal Medicine*
> (*ca.* 2ND CENTURY BC)

Following some of the nutritional recommendations, practising the touch therapies and exercises for body and mind, will enhance your knowledge of how to stay well. Start to trust and develop your own intuition or instinct, while continuing to seek advice wherever it can be found: your GP's surgery, with a homoeopath, a healer, nutritionist, reflexologist, acupuncturist, aromatherapist, etc. or someone skilled in many aspects of natural healthcare; and with your own 'inner doctor', who knows what is best for you. *Never* under-estimate the body's own healing mechanism: it is extremely powerful and can reverse and repair most of the body's disharmonies, given the right conditions.

Self-knowledge and personal changes of this nature take both time and patience, but by following this holistic approach, the effects will be more powerful and longer lasting as they take into account the close interrelationship between your mind, body and spirit. I hope that by reading this book you will be able to learn a great deal about yourself and experience the wonder and wisdom of the Chinese system of medicine. Your body is prepared to tell you what is going on with it, if you are prepared to listen, feel and observe.

Jennifer Harper
February 1997

Past and Present

'Vis medicatrix naturae' – the 'healing power of nature' is the foundation on which the majority of therapies that come under the heading of 'alternative' or 'complementary' medicine are based. Nature cure or naturopathy is a system of health-orientated medicine which recognizes that the body has an inherent ability to heal itself and is a way of life which advocates living according to natural principles. Twenty-five centuries ago, Hippocrates believed that patients could often heal themselves by employing proper procedures and thus they had considerable responsibility for their health.

> *Health is the expression of a harmonious balance between various components of man's nature, the environment and ways of life ... nature is the physician of disease.*
>
> HIPPOCRATES

In the 17th century, the Hippocratic doctrine was superseded by a new approach that was soon to embody the philosophy of modern medicine as we know it today. René Descartes introduced the 'analytical' model and because it was so radically different, ultimately the principles underlying modern medicine came to be referred to as 'Cartesian'. The Cartesian approach separated the mind from the body and consequently the work of natural physicians went into decline. Chemistry and analysis dominated thinking and medicine began its retreat away from nature. This new philosophy embodied the principle that if plants contained simple, effective compounds then why not make a synthetic version of the active ingredients and bypass nature altogether? The emphasis of medicine changed from supporting the body's power to heal itself by restoring balance to the mind, body and spirit to one where the body was reduced to structural parts such as organs, tissues and cells.

The physician in his new role was able to separate the whole into individual parts in an attempt to discern the function of each component; the offending 'diseased' component could therefore be isolated and removed by surgical intervention or treated by the use of medication. However, this restricted outlook has limited the scope and effectiveness of medicine as it has tended to equate the cure of disease with the control of symptoms. Perhaps here we should reflect on the wise words once spoken by the Greek philosopher Plato:

> The cure of any part should not be attempted without treatment of the whole. No attempt should be made to cure the body without the soul and if the head and body are to be healthy you must begin by curing the mind, for this is the great error of our day in the treatment of the human body that physicians first separate the soul from the body.

Today, however, we are experiencing a resurgence in the popularity of natural methods and holistic techniques where the aim is to restore and promote balance in the 'whole' person. Until relatively recently, it had been viewed that allopathic (orthodox) medicine was incompatible with 'alternative' therapies. However, we are swiftly moving towards finding a place where both sides can work together in a fully integrated system of healthcare. The World Health Organization's goal is 'health for all by the year 2000'. Perhaps by that time we will have created a system which recognizes that physical, bio-chemical, psychological, spiritual and environmental factors all play a part in governing the state of our health; a system which respects and accepts the diversity, individuality and potential of each human and where the ultimate aim is to restore equilibrium to all levels of our being and sustain it.

PART I

Chinese Medicine

Chinese medicine is a system of diagnosis and healthcare which has evolved over the last 4,000 years and is a unique approach to understanding the human body. In Chinese medicine, health is viewed as a totally complete state of well-being, which is a different approach to Western medicine, which defines health as merely the 'absence of disease'. The *Huang Ti Nei Jing*, or *Yellow Emperor's Classic of Internal Medicine*, is a corpus of writings on Chinese Medicine. There are several versions, some of which no longer exist. The most commonly known was compiled by Wang Ping during the Tang dynasty. It was an intellectual tradition which started in the 2nd–3rd centuries BC. It was considered then, as it is today, to be an indispensable treatise on acupuncture, and an important reference material for the study and practice of Traditional Chinese Medicine (TCM). While back in the 2nd century BC it reflected current beliefs and practices, it also claimed to draw on ancient sources dating back a further 3,000 years when people were said to have experienced high levels of health and greater longevity.

TCM is based on the belief that all humanity is part of the natural environment and that health or balance can only be achieved when one follows the natural law, adapting to the changes of the seasons and the surrounding environment. This is the philosophy of the *dao*, which was an essential way of life before even the *Huang Ti Nei Jing* had been written. The Chinese believed (and still do today) that the more we stray from living in harmony with the *dao*, the more certain it is that no form of external medicine or treatment could ever compensate for the stresses that will affect mind, body and spirit. The theories of *yin* and *yang*, together with the notion of the five elements, were developed through ancient Chinese rituals of observing nature's ever changing cycles. These theories are fundamental to Chinese medicine.

The Five Elements or Phases

It is thought that Tsou Yen was the official creator of the doctrine of the five elements (though technically the correct translation from the Chinese would be the five 'movements' or 'phases'). The five elements are Wood, Fire, Earth, Metal and Water. These are related to the different seasons of the year and to organs in the human body. By knowing and understanding these elements or phases, we can discover how to balance the extremes of each season and comprehend what unique opportunities for growth arise with each. The organs are interlinked with the seasons, temperatures, colours and tastes, to name but a few associations, all of which have some relevance to our health and well-being.

The Wood phase occurs in Spring, which is a time in nature of activity and new beginnings. This is followed by the Fire element in Summer, which is the season of abundance where the ideas that were put into action in the Spring have blossomed and flowered. The Earth phase arrives in late Summer and is the harvest season, a time when we can reap the benefits of the seeds planted in the early Spring. Metal is connected with Autumn, the time of decline when nature slowly begins to withdraw in preparation for the Winter. The life force in nature lies dormant during the Winter months of the Water element, like the latent seed that is lying still and waiting to burst open in the Spring to begin the cycle once again. (*See table on page 20.*)

Sheng and Ko Cycles

The five elements are often depicted as illustrated in the diagram opposite, which shows how the organs are all interrelated and can demonstrate how an imbalance in one element will have a corresponding effect on the other elements within the cycle. There are two important cycles in the five element theory: the *Sheng*, or generation cycle, and the *Ko*, or controlling cycle.

Generation, or Sheng Cycle
Qi (or life-force) travels round from element to element:

- *Water* nourishes the plants and trees, generating *Wood*.
- *Wood* can be burned to generate *Fire*.
- *Fire* leaves behind ashes that are absorbed into the *Earth*.
- *Earth* contains the ores that form *Metal*.
- *Metal* (mineral ores) enrich the *Water*.

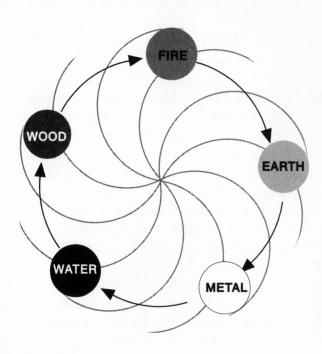

The Sheng cycle

There is another way of interpreting this cycle, which is to substitute the elements for the key organs (these are known in Chinese medicine as the *yin* organs). So, when Water nourishes Wood, the kidney, which is the *yin* organ of the Water element, helps to feed the liver and strengthen its energy. By strengthening the liver (Wood), blood is generated which is stored in this organ. Blood is needed by the *yin* organ of the Fire element, the heart, so the liver plays a supporting role to the heart. The fiery energy of the heart supports the spleen, the *yin* organ of the Earth element, by supplying the necessary heat and energy to assist the spleen in its function of processing food. The spleen then nurtures Metal by taking the resultant food essence upwards and combining this with the air from the lungs to form pure *qi*. The lungs, the yin organ of the Metal element, then play a supporting role to the kidneys by sending moist *qi* or energy to be stored in the kidneys. Diseases where there is weakness or 'deficiency' (as it is known in TCM) tend to follow the path of the *Sheng* cycle, where the weak 'child' draws heavily on its 'mother' for support, so draining her reserves.

Mother and Child Relationship

This is sometimes expressed as the law of the Mother and Child. One way to interpret this is to imagine a simple family scenario. When a mother has a baby and breastfeeds her, if there are any illnesses with the mother, it affects the quality of her milk. This then will have a corresponding effect on the child, who will become sick as she is not receiving adequate nutrition. The other possibility with this law is that the child could be particularly hungry and so deplete the mother by drawing too heavily on her supplies, leading to the mother becoming ill. The mother's role is to ensure that the child's and her own vital needs are met.

Building the organs into the picture, a good example to use is the liver as the mother and the heart as the child. When the 'mother' (the liver) is sick, it will affect the flow of *qi* to the 'child' (the heart). This means that the 'child' could start to produce symptoms such as palpitations, anxiety and chest pains.

Frequently in Western medicine, the first reaction is to treat the immediate obvious symptoms of disease. However, if we could only look a little further and find out *why* the body has produced symptoms, then perhaps we could learn to treat the cause of the problem instead of merely its symptoms. This is the importance of understanding where the 'mother' of a disease lies. In the example given above, treating the heart alone would not be the most suitable route to take, as the original cause in this instance stems from the liver. By treating the true cause of the imbalance, you will re-establish harmony in all the related organs.

Chart of mother and child relationships

Mother	Child
Wood (liver)	Fire (heart)
Fire (heart)	Earth (spleen)
Earth (spleen)	Metal (lungs)
Metal (lungs)	Water (kidneys)
Water (kidneys)	Wood (liver)

Controlling, or Ko Cycle

The controlling or *Ko* cycle applies constraints to the relationships between various elements:

- *Wood* can deplete the *Earth* of its nutrients.
- *Earth* absorbs *Water*, channelling and containing it.
- *Water* can overcome *Fire*.
- *Fire* can melt *Metal*.
- *Metal* controls *Wood* (as metal tools can cut through trees).

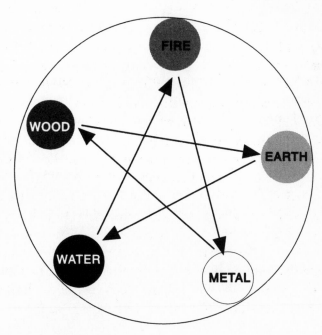

The Ko cycle

In organ terms, we may see a disease beginning, for example, in the Wood element (the liver). If the problem goes undetected, it will affect the spleen and digestion (Earth), which then go on to imbalance the kidney (Water). The next element in the *Ko* cycle is Fire, so we see the disharmony going on to affect the heart and then the lung (Metal). It is interesting to note the correlation of the heart and kidneys when the *Ko* cycle follows a destructive path: this is confirmed in Western medicine when excessive fluid retention weakens the heart and diuretics are prescribed.

The five element theory shows the interrelationship of the organs and phases in a very general way. There are other interpretations of the cycles, but the above are the most popular and accepted theories. However, it is essential to understand that the relationships between the different organs can be very complex. Sometimes it may be that one element is out of balance, but when the disease is chronic it is very likely that all of the key organs will be affected to a greater or lesser degree. There will still be a major cause or 'mother' of the illness, but some organs may have developed a hyperactive or excess pattern in response to the illness and others may be showing signs of deficiency (*see page 11, Excess and Deficiency*).

Yin and Yang

Traditional Chinese medicine holds that the material world is in a constant state of flux due to the movement of *yin* and *yang*, two opposing elements which are mutually dependent (that is, they cannot exist without one another). The theory of *yin* and *yang* is used to help explain the physiological imbalances and any pathological changes in the human body. The resulting information is then used for diagnostic purposes. *Yin*, translated literally, means the 'dark side of the mountain' and represents qualities such as darkness, coldness, stillness, etc. *Yang* is translated as the 'bright side of the mountain', representing light, warmth and activity. In the chart opposite, *yin* and *yang* are broken down here into four categories which can help to clarify and illustrate some of the roles these two opposites play in life.

YANG	YIN

In nature

Spring/Summer	Autumn/Winter
East/South	West/North
Day	Night
Hot	Cold
Fire	Water
Light	Dark
Sun	Moon

In our bodies

Male	Female
Energy	Blood
Surfaces of the body	Internal parts of the body
Back of the body	Front of the body
Upper body	Lower body
Right side of the body	Left side of the body

In ill-health

Acute symptoms	Chronic disease
Heat and high temperature	Cold and low temperature
Dryness	Moistness

Organs/meridians

Gallbladder	Liver
Small intestine	Heart
Stomach	Spleen
Large intestine	Lungs
Bladder	Kidneys
triple warmer	*pericardium*

The Eight Principles

There are four opposing diagnostic considerations in Traditional Chinese Medicine which help the practitioner to understand the true nature of a disease or imbalance:

1. Interior and exterior
2. Heat and cold
3. Excess and deficiency
4. Yin and yang

There are many combinations of these patterns, which are too complex to explain in detail in a book of this nature. However, we can look briefly at each individual pairing:

Interior and exterior patterns can help to explain the aetiology of an illness – in other words, where it has come from and where in the body it actually resides. Interior diseases may be of an emotional origin (that is, caused by prolonged grief, fear, anger, etc.) and tend to develop slowly. They are more chronic and long-standing than exterior illnesses. An exterior disease tends to be more of an acute nature, brought on by external causes known as the 'six pernicious influences': Heat, Summer Heat, Dryness, Wind, Cold and Damp. You will see later in this book that these influences are connected with the elements and organs. For example, too much cold can injure the kidney/Water element, too much heat can injure the heart/Fire element (*see table on page 20*). If the body and *qi* are strong, you are less likely to be susceptible to these external influences. However, when there is an imbalance in the body and a weakness or deficiency of *qi*, you are more likely to contract an illness.

Heat and cold are used primarily to describe whether the body has symptoms of either a 'cold' nature – for example, low body temperature, pale complexion, pale urine, loose stools and a desire for hot drinks and a warm environment – or a 'hot' nature – the person will very often feel hot, look red in the face, have a thirst for cold liquids, crave fresh air or cold temperatures, and have dark urine and constipation. This information will guide the practitioner towards a suitable treatment: for example, someone showing symptoms of a cold nature will be prescribed warming herbs and warming foods. Raw foods and cold liquids would not be deemed suitable for illnesses of this nature, as the stomach has to warm the cold food, using up more *qi* to digest it and ultimately weakening the individual further.

Excess and deficiency is an extremely important differentiation in Chinese medicine and can demonstrate the impact that an illness is having on the body. If the patient is already weak, then he or she is likely to exhibit further deficiency symptoms (such as fatigue, loss of appetite, a soft voice and lassitude). Conversely, someone showing signs of excess will display hyper- or over-activity of body functions, such as heavy breathing and a loud voice. As the latter type is ultimately stronger, he or she will have sufficient *qi* to generate a strong reaction to the pathogen and is therefore more likely to present more obvious, visible symptoms. The important point to be made here is that the 'excess' patient may show more marked signs of illness, but the 'deficient' patient may be in a more critical state, and care must be taken to ensure that he or she does not become weakened further.

Yin and *yang*, as discussed earlier, are fundamental to TCM. They encompass the six influences above: your practitioner when making a diagnosis will check to see what imbalances you have and whether they could be defined as interior or exterior, hot or cold, excess or deficient. This will help the practitioner to understand and determine the *yin/yang* disharmony in your body.

Essential Substances

There are various substances that are considered to be essential in Chinese medicine which help to nourish all levels of our being. I have outlined below the five fundamental substances: *Jing* (essence), *Shen* (spirit), *Xue* (blood), *Qi* (life-force) and *Jin Ye* (body fluids).

Jing

We are all born with this special prenatal essence or *Jing* which we inherit from our parents and which, in many respects, helps to define our basic constitution. Children born of healthy parents will have a strong essence or *Jing*, whereas children whose parents have a weaker constitution will often have inherited less. *Jing* is discussed in more depth in the chapter on the kidneys (*page 129*), as the kidneys store the *Jing*.

Shen

The *Shen* or spirit resides in the heart which, according to the principles of Chinese medicine, is often seen as the organ most connected with heaven. The concept of the *Shen* is a complex one, as there are many interpretations. It is probably best translated as 'spirit', although some authorities interpret it as the mind. More information on the *Shen* is found in the chapter on the heart (*page 81*).

Xue

The blood (*Xue*) plays a vital role in both Western and Chinese medicine. The Chinese believe that blood travels not only in the blood vessels, but also in the meridians or energy channels of the body. It is classified as a *yin* substance.

Qi

Qi or *chi* (pronounced 'chee') can be translated as 'vital energy' or life-force, but even these words do not capture what *qi* really is. It has been described as the force that nourishes both the body and mind, and the free-flow of this vital energy around the body is seen as imperative to our health and wellbeing. If the *qi* becomes imbalanced, or there is a blockage (*stagnation*), there is too little (a *deficiency*) or even too much (*excess*), disease can result. The flow of this vital energy can be impeded by poor diet, lack of exercise, poor breathing and posture, scar tissue and psychological stress.

Qi flows through the body in pathways called *meridians*.

Jin Ye

Jin Ye pertains to all the other body fluids and secretions – saliva, synovial fluid (lubricates the joints) and mucus. Oedema (water retention) illustrates an imbalance in body fluids.

The Meridian System

The meridians are channels that carry the *qi* around the body. There are 12 major organ meridians and eight extra channels. Both acupuncture and acupressure work on specific points along the meridians called acupuncture points. If these are congested it can impede the energy flow, possibly resulting in pain or problems in the associated organ. Working on chosen points on the meridian can help to circulate the energy and rebalance the body.

Pericardium and Triple Warmer

The Chinese include two other meridians, the *pericardium* and the *triple warmer/burner*. These are not organs in the physical sense, but have very important roles to play in health. The *pericardium* is known as the 'heart protector' whose key function is to stop anything harmful from reaching the heart. It is thought to take the brunt of physical and emotional pressure.

The *triple warmer* (*san jiao*) is the method by which the *Jin Ye* or body fluids move from one organ function to another. Another interpretation maintains that the *triple warmer* regulates the temperature of the internal organs, ensuring they are kept within their ideal range. It is the only channel which traverses the body in a spiral fashion, rather than a straight line.

The *triple warmer* is divided into three sections: the upper warmer, which consists of the lungs, heart and *pericardium*; the middle warmer, which consists of the digestive organs; and the lower warmer, which contains the remaining organs of elimination as well as the kidneys and liver. However, some TCM practitioners consider the liver to be in the middle warmer.

The Organs

All the major organs in the body are paired according to the principles of *yin* and *yang*, as in the chart (*page 8*), and with one of the five elements. The *yin* organs are also called the 'zang' organs; they are solid organs involved primarily with collecting and storing, whereas the *yang* or 'fu' organs are hollow, more involved in transforming and transporting. When disharmony affecting the organs is brought back into balance as much as possible, diseases of the mind and body subside.

Tongue and Pulse Diagnosis

These two diagnostic techniques play a fundamental role in Traditional Chinese Medicine. It is not appropriate to describe either method in depth here, as they have to be carried out by a trained practitioner. Suffice to say that pulse diagnosis bears no resemblance to the physical examination of the pulse carried out in Western medicine; the latter is primarily concerned with the speed of the pulse. TCM focuses on the quality of the pulse in six different positions, three positions on each wrist at a superficial or deep levels. Acupuncturists also can detect imbalances from a medial position. The *yin* organs are felt at a deep position and the *yang* organs at the superficial level. On the left wrist you find the heart, liver and kidney at the deep level and their *yang* counterpart organs, small intestine, gallbladder and bladder, at the superficial level. The right pulses denote the lung, spleen and *pericardium yin* organs and superficial positions reflect the large intestine, stomach and *triple warmer*.

In tongue diagnosis, a practitioner assesses the condition of the tongue, observing in particular the colour, texture (wet, dry, shiny, sticky, etc.), shape and any coating on the body of the tongue. These characteristics may vary in different sections of the tongue, which correspond to the organs of the body.

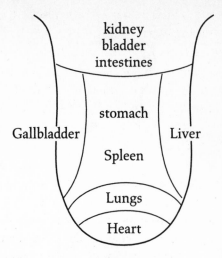

kidney
bladder
intestines

stomach

Gallbladder

Liver

Spleen

Lungs

Heart

Tongue diagnosis

Moxibustion

Moxibustion is the process of burning the herb Mugwort (Moxa) over certain areas of the body (including acupressure points) to increase internal warmth and energy both in the meridians and throughout the body. Mugwort (*Artemisia vulgaris latiflora*) has the ability to transfer heat generated by burning a moxa stick approximately 2.5 cm away from the desired location on the body. It is an excellent preventative as well as a tonic, as it regulates, nourishes and moves the *qi* and can also warm it if we are cold. Burning Moxa over acupressure point Stomach 36 is an excellent way of increasing energy – the Chinese recommend that everyone over 30 does this (*see page 58*). Burning it over Bladder 23 also increases energy and supports the kidneys (*see page 124*). If there is no movement or warmth in the lower burner, it is good to burn moxa over points CV 4 and 6 (*see diagram overleaf*).

CV 4 (below) and 6 (above)

At the *very* first signs of a cold or flu, moxa LI 4 (*see page 211*) for five minutes, on each hand – this will help stop the cold or flu from developing, but only if done immediately you feel the symptoms coming on.

WARNING: Never use moxibustion on an area where there is a lot of heat or congestion. Other contraindications include fever, high blood pressure, diabetes or sensitive skin.

Technique

Moxa is best applied by using a moxa stick, which looks rather like a large cigar (can be purchased from a Chinese pharmacy). Peel the top coloured wrapper and light the stick, allowing it to burn until it produces some smoke. Holding the stick like a pencil with your hand halfway up its length, place the burning tip approximately 2.5 cm above the chosen acupressure point or area. Feel the warmth increasing – when it becomes too hot, withdraw the stick for a few moments. Briefly touch the point with your hand to cool the skin, then reapply the heat using a 'pecking' technique: hold the tip close until you cannot tolerate any more heat, then pull it away. Alternatively, you can move the stick slowly in a clockwise direction over the affected area. Continue for several minutes until you feel that the heat has truly penetrated the area and warmed it up. To extinguish, cut off the oxygen to the stick by stubbing it out in a jar of salt or sand, or wrap it in foil, or place it upside down into a long metal candlestick holder (never hold it under water).

Emotions

Every phase (of the five phases) has specific emotions associated with it. Extremes of emotions can have a negative impact on the organs, just as an imbalanced organ can have a profound effect on the state of our emotions.

Earth
Worry or sympathy are the emotions connected to the Earth element. Sympathy can display itself at times when we are over-sympathetic to circumstances or, alternatively, cannot bear people fussing over us. Someone who continually seeks as much sympathy as possible, the individual who happily tells you all about their health problems and woes, or who is constantly worrying, has an imbalance in the spleen or stomach.

Wood
Excessive amounts of anger or feelings of frustration, irritation or suppressed rage point to the Wood element and show us that it is not functioning harmoniously. The Chinese, however, readily admit there are appropriate times for expressing anger and it is better to vent our feelings rather than to seethe and suppress this powerful emotion.

Fire
Laughter and joy are valuable emotions and today there is sadly not enough of these wonderful emotions on display. Someone who can't laugh or show love and affection, or who demonstrates excess amounts, reveals a Fire imbalance.

Water

Fear is a very real emotion and without it we might not realize when we are in dangerous situations. It can, however, consume us and this is when it is damaging to the Water element.

Metal

Finally, grief too is an important emotion that we experience when we go through the loss of something special. If there is an imbalance in the Metal element, the grieving process can be prolonged beyond its natural term.

Lifestyle

Our lifestyle and its effects on our health are very important factors in Chinese medicine, especially in the areas of diet, exercise and sexual activity. Diet is an important factor in most cultures and the Chinese are no different, as a quote in the *Nei Jing* illustrates: *'When essence is deficient, replenish it with food.'* Chinese diets are, in a sense, more holistic and primarily designed to heal many common ailments, from constipation and diarrhoea to colds or skin disorders. The Chinese approach is far more complete than the Western one, as it dates back to the time before foods were classified according to their protein, fat, carbohydrate and nutrient content. The Chinese focused on the different qualities and primary actions of foods which were used to help create balance in the body. This system is known as food energetics; according to this system, all foods have specific qualities and effects on the body.

Exercise is an important factor, but it is a matter of balance: moderate exercise gets the *qi* flowing in the body but excessive amounts drain our vital kidney energy and can weaken the body. Understanding the concepts of duality and of balancing rest with activity is essential. According to TCM, too much sex can weaken the body thus reducing our vitality and energy levels. This is explained in greater depth under the chapter on the kidney (*page 129*).

Body Clock

Every organ in the body has a two-hour period of maximum activity which means that when the organ is in its natural time period, it has greater energy than the others. If we honoured these times and let them guide us in our activities we would be much healthier. If you find that you have a dip in energy or feel worse at a particular time of day, then this could be pointing to the particular organ which falls into that time period. For example, the stomach is in power between 7 and 9 a.m. This is the time that digestion is at its peak. Therefore, the old advice 'Breakfast like a King, lunch like a Prince and dine like a Pauper' is in fact quite correct, as breakfast is the time of the day when the body digests foods best. If you feel particularly tired between 5 and 7 p.m. in the evening, your kidney energy may not be as strong as it should be. If you can't get to sleep between the hours of 11 p.m. and 3 a.m., then your Wood element is out of balance and needs treatment.

Early Signs of Disease

The wonder of the Chinese system of medicine is that changes often begin to occur approximately six to nine months *before* a disease arises. We can pick up on the particular stress signals that nature is providing if we can understand more about the body and know what signs to look out for. The body can show imbalances in a variety of ways: a hatred or passion for a particular season of the year, a love of a particular colour or a desire to avoid wearing a specific colour, or even a change in the colour of your face. Your body will emit a specific odour when an organ becomes imbalanced, and your emotions will change (since the organs in the body influence our emotions). By understanding and listening to your body, you can find out why it is functioning the way it is and then take the necessary steps towards improving your health.

The table overleaf charts the traditional Chinese interpretations given to each of the five elements and its related organs.

Five Elements Table

	Wood	Fire	Earth	Metal	Water
Direction	East	South	Centre	West	North
Colour	Green	Red	Yellow	White	Blue/Black
Climate	Wind	Heat	Humidity	Dryness	Cold
Season	Spring	Summer	Late Summer	Autumn	Winter
Yin Organ	Liver	Heart	Spleen	Lungs	Kidneys
Time	1–3 a.m.	11a.m.–1 p.m.	9–11 a.m.	3–5 a.m.	5–7 p.m.
Yang Organ	Gallbladder	Small Intestine	Stomach	Large Intestine	Bladder
Time	11 p.m.–1 a.m.	1–3 p.m.	7–9 a.m. /	5–7a.m. /	3–5 p.m.
Stage	Birth	Growth	Transformation	Absorption	Storage
Number	8	7	5	9	6
Planet	Jupiter	Mars	Saturn	Venus	Mercury
Spirit	Hun	Shen	Yi	P'o	Zhi
Body Tissue	Tendons/Ligaments	Blood Vessels	Muscles/Flesh	Skin	Bones/Marrow
Voice Sound	Shouting	Laughter	Singing	Weeping	Moaning
Emotion	Anger	Joy	Worry/Sympathy	Grief	Fear
Taste	Sour	Bitter	Sweet	Spicy	Salty
Odour	Rancid	Burnt	Fragrant	Pungent	Putrid
Sense Organ	Eyes	Tongue	Mouth	Nose	Ears
Reflector	Nails	Complexion	Lips	Body Hair	Head Hair
Secretion	Tears	Perspiration	Saliva	Nasal Discharge	Sputum

NB The time for the *pericardium* is 7–9 p.m.; for the *triple warmer*, 9–11 p.m.

PART II

The Therapies

This section explains the background of the therapies included in *Body Wisdom*: what they are and how they work, together with general guidelines and information on relevant techniques.

I have chosen a cross-section of natural therapies that I combine in my own clinic as I believe that the greatest results are gained by working with a variety of healing techniques to nourish and support weak organs and body systems.

Please note that although I have separated the organs (Part III) into individual chapters to make them easier to understand, it is important to remember that these organs and body systems are completely interconnected and must not be seen as isolated structures – they are part of the 'whole'.

Chinese Nutrition

What Is Chinese Nutrition?
Diet is important to most cultures and the Chinese traditional view on nutrition is no different. Food is considered to have very potent healing properties or energies. Diets are traditionally holistic and designed to heal many common ailments ranging from the common cold to skin disorders.

How It Works
Traditional Chinese Medicine teaches that certain foods and flavours act on the 10 internal organs; some foods have a positive effect on more than one organ. Carrot, for example, works on

both the lungs and spleen; celery works on the stomach and the kidneys. This basic relationship between the internal organs and flavours has been studied over many years; the Chinese tradition believes that a combination of five flavours ensures balance, harmony and vitality in the body. Foods also have different properties – for example, cool, warm, dry or damp – and too much of any one food can have adverse effects. For example, warming foods are considered to raise the metabolic rate and cooling foods to lower it … an interesting fact as most Western diet books focus on raw (cold) foods such as fruit and salads for weight loss!

Pungent foods act on the Metal element. Examples include green onions, chives, cloves, parsley and coriander. Their main action is to induce perspiration and stimulate circulation.

Sweet foods act on the Earth element. Examples include cherries, bananas, honey, sugar and watermelon. They slow down acute symptoms and neutralize the toxic effects of other foods.

Sour foods act on the Wood element. They include lemons, rhubarb and plums. They can help with diarrhoea and excessive perspiration.

Bitter foods act on the Fire element. Examples include seaweed, bitter lettuce, coffee, asparagus and kelp. They influence the heart and small intestine, can reduce body heat, eliminate excess body fluids and induce diarrhoea.

Salty foods act on the Water element. They include salt, seaweeds and kelp, and affect the kidneys and bladder.

General Dietary Guidelines

Choosing the correct foods and dietary programme will always be an individual matter, but there are various guidelines that can start you off on the right track.

1. Try to eat meals in the right frame of mind, in other words, don't sit down to a meal if you are feeling angry or frustrated. Being calm and relaxed while you eat is almost as important as the food you consume. A peaceful state of mind aids digestion and assimilation of all the nutrients in the foods you eat. Using all your senses when you eat the meal, such as smelling the food, visually enjoying the look of your meal and tasting it, means that the body will be far more prepared to absorb the food.

2. Chew your food properly, as starch digestion begins in the mouth. Chewing your food also means that you take more time to eat the meal and, therefore, the body will have time to tell you when it is getting full. Rushing food down, as is common practice in today's society, means that we do not recognize the 'full' sign until we have gone past it!

3. Cut down on coffee, tea, alcohol, fried/fatty foods, refined convenience products and sweets.

4. Increase your consumption of water. If the weather is cold, make sure that the water you drink is slightly warmed (at least room temperature) rather than ice cold. Cold water can cause the stomach to contract.

5. Eat whatever grows locally, and according to the seasons. Nature has given us the ideal foods to cope with each temperature and season. Eating salads in Winter is not ideal (unless you have had a warming meal prior to this), just as you probably wouldn't choose to have carrot and turnip stew on a hot Summer's day! The current trend focuses on eating foods as raw as possible. However, in the Chinese tradition, too much raw or 'cold' food in the diet is known to extinguish the 'digestive fires'. Too much cold food may lead to a 'damp spleen', which can give rise to symptoms such as oedema, weight gain, loose stools and abdominal bloating.

6. Do not eat late in the evening. At this time the body is naturally going into a 'rest' phase and cannot digest food properly. It is far better to eat a good breakfast when the stomach is in power (between 7 and 9 a.m.) and digestion is at its peak.

7. Eat whole foods and organic produce where possible. Pesticides and chemicals used in modern farming practices are very harmful to the immune system and liver. If you have no

choice, wash produce in either cider vinegar and water, or salt water. There are also manufactured products available from health shops which are designed to eliminate agricultural residues.

8. When cooking grains and pulses, soak them overnight in filtered water with a little vinegar and a piece of kombu seaweed. Discard the liquid and cook them in fresh water. This process will break down the compounds that can cause gas and also increase the nutritional value and digestibility of the food.

9. Avoid cooking with nonstick pans, aluminium and copper, as these materials can leach metals into the food. Stainless steel, glass or earthenware are better choices.

10. Avoid food that has been either irradiated or microwaved.

Foods

- There is a lot of new research coming out in the US which suggests that we are not eating sufficient protein due to an obsession with low-fat and high-carbohydrate diets. Ensure that you are getting enough protein. Buy organic meats wherever possible and keep to lean cuts – and remember, fresh fish is always preferable to frozen. Also, avoid fish from very polluted waters. Seeds (*see below*) are a good source of non-meat proteins.

- Increase your consumption of vegetables, but not raw ones when you are first making changes to your normal diet. This is because raw foods are very good cleansers, and if the body is very toxic the cleansing reaction will be too powerful. It is best to start gently, so eat plenty of home-made vegetable soups, lightly steamed vegetables and stir-fries.

- Stir-frying is an excellent way of cooking vegetables as the nutrients are sealed within and you can include wonderful fresh herbs such as garlic, ginger, coriander and fenugreek sprouts. It is best not to use oil, however, as fats when heated change chemically and are not very good for the liver. Instead, use a little boiling water, then start by sweating garlic, onions and ginger. When these have released some moisture, add more spices and then finally your vegetables.

- Sprouting sesame, pumpkin and sunflower seeds increases their nutritional value so they become real 'superfoods'. These three seeds combined produce protein, but remember to chew them particularly well to ensure that your body will utilize and assimilate them readily. Sprinkle onto porridge, soups, stir-fries, etc. Other foods to sprout include mung and aduki beans, alfalfa and chick peas. Leslie Kenton's books have a lot of information on sprouting and include useful tables illustrating the length of sprouting times for different seeds.

- Cut down on acidic grains such as wheat and rye and start including more wholegrain brown rice, millet and quinoa in your diet. If your digestion is weak, include white basmati rice, as wholegrain brown rice can be difficult to digest for some people. Millet is an alkaline grain which helps cleanse the body and lower acid levels. Quinoa, the mother food of the Incas, is very high in protein. All these are excellent cleansing foods, which are at the same time very gentle on the system.
- Raw, cold-pressed virgin seed oils are an excellent addition to the diet and can be mixed into a fresh salad dressing, thus adding essential fatty acids to the diet.
- Keep your saturated fat intake as low as you can: grill foods and follow the boiling water method of cooking outlined earlier.
- It is also best to avoid citrus fruits such as oranges as they are known as 'aggressive' cleansers, and if your liver is not as strong as it should be, it may experience difficulty breaking down the fruit acids. Oranges are known to increase mucus levels in the body. The Chinese believe that too much fruit in Winter is not to be recommended as it does not grow naturally at this time of the year.
- When the weather is warm, more salad foods can be included in your diet. In Winter, a small salad can be eaten at the end of your meal if desired. Use good quality oils, ideally cold-pressed virgin olive oil mixed with apple cider vinegar to make up a dressing for the salad (include fresh garlic if you can!).
- Herb teas and drinks such as Caro, Barley Cup or Bambu can be consumed, but have them without cow's milk or sugar. If you are a tea drinker, try Chinese Green tea. This contains antioxidants and the caffeine levels are lower and far less concentrated than those found in black tea. However, it should still be consumed in moderation!

Breakfast

- Breakfast could be oatmeal porridge, preferably using organic oats and apple juice or water, not milk, to moisten.
- Milk is difficult to digest and contains hormones, steroids and antibiotics. Dairy foods increase the production of mucus in the body, and a large number of people cannot efficiently digest these foods. I consider the best alternatives to be almond milk, rice milk, oat milk, sheep and goat's milk.

Lunch

- Lunch could consist of a home-made vegetable soup or brown rice with vegetables. If you follow a food combining programme (*see Further Reading, page 217*), then the above is fine, or if you want a protein meal, exchange the rice for a protein dish of your choice.

Dinner

- Dinner could be a repeat of the above, or a stir-fry with fresh organic vegetables and either millet, rice or quinoa. Again, protein can be added to the meal. It is a good idea to soak any of the grains used for between 12 and 24 hours, as this increases their nutritional value and makes them easier to assimilate in the body. It is best to restrict your intake of puddings; if necessary, nibble on unsulphured dried fruit that has been soaked in mineral water for several hours.

Exercise

Exercise is viewed in very different lights by Chinese and Western societies. Qigong and T'ai Chi are the main forms in China, and are recognized as invaluable aids to ensuring that the energy system is balanced and strong. It is thought that the Chinese were involved in these forms of exercise even before the birth of acupuncture. Gentle to moderate amounts of exercise are recommended to keep the blood and *qi* (*see page 12*) circulating. Not taking any exercise at all can lead to sluggishness and stagnation, which the Chinese see as encouraging the onset of many illnesses. Strenuous exercise is not endorsed, especially at certain times of the year as it is considered to deplete the body and kidney *qi*. For example, when the body energy is at its lowest point during the Winter season, gentle forms of exercise such as walking and swimming are enough to stimulate and encourage the circulatory system to be free-flowing and, at the same time, not drain our vital inner reserves. (*For more on this, see the chapters on organs connected to Winter: the bladder and kidneys, pages 114 and 129.*)

In the chapters on specific organs of the body, stretches are included that will help to improve the flow of *qi* along the relevant meridians, so enhancing organ function. Suppleness in the muscles, like in a new sapling, is a sign of a healthy liver (*see page 163*), whereas stiffness and difficulty stretching can indicate that there is stagnation and an imbalance within the organ.

Reflexology

What Is Reflexology?

Reflexology, or reflex zone therapy as it is sometimes called, works on the principle that all the organs and systems of the body are reflected on the soles and the backs of the feet. The body is divided into 10 zones (corresponding to the 10 fingers and toes) which run up the entire length of the body, five on each side. The right side of the body corresponds with the right foot, the left side of the body with the left foot. 'Twin' organs such as the lungs and kidneys have reflex points on each foot; the colon starts on the right foot and, just as the transverse colon travels horizontally across the body, so the reflex travels across from the right foot to the left foot. When specific reflex points are stimulated, these reflexes increase circulation in different parts of the body, healing, nourishing and energizing the corresponding organs.

The origin of a pressure-point system in the feet can be found some 3,000 years ago in China; the system then spread to India and Tibet. Native tribes in North America also understood the relationship between reflex points and the internal organs, and so practised this therapy based on their knowledge. In China this was superseded by acupressure and acupuncture. Reflexology arrived in Europe in the early part of the 20th century and was developed by Dr William Fitzgerald, who noticed that by applying pressure to certain parts of the body, an analgesic effect could be produced on a corresponding area. Together with Dr Edward Bowers, he produced a book in 1916 called *Zone Therapy* – and so founded the subject as we know it today. Eunice Ingham developed the theory further by concentrating more on the feet, calling this the 'Ingham method of compression massage'. Today she is known as the founder of foot reflexology.

How It Works

There are many explanations suggesting how reflexology actually works. Certain theories connect it to the nervous system, as there are about 72,000 nerve endings in the feet. It is thought that 'crystals', or waste products that the body has not effectively eliminated, are deposited in the feet. Massaging the appropriate reflex points can help to disperse and dissolve these crystals. These are then removed by the lymphatic system and eliminated from the body. It is also thought that reflexology can help to clear energy blockages in the meridians, the pathways of energy which spread throughout the body like an intricate web (*these are discussed further under the Acupressure section opposite*).

Techniques

The thumb-walking technique is one of the most popular and easiest for the lay person to understand. All you need to do is press your thumb on the reflexology point, then bend the thumb at the first joint to 'walk' it along the whole reflex area, feeling for any 'crystals' or hard, granular lumps. Small circular movements directly over certain reflexes also help to disperse any of these 'gritty' areas that may have formed in the foot. Talc is one of the best mediums to work with; you can finish by massaging the whole area using a base oil (olive, sunflower, apricot, almond) with a few drops of your chosen essential oils.

In Chinese medicine, the feet are very important in terms of the many acupuncture points that begin on the feet. Therefore, it is highly beneficial after working on specific reflexes in the foot to give the whole foot a massage, paying special attention to the area between the toes and the tips of the toes.

General guidelines

1. Never overstimulate a reflex point. Working on an area for approximately one minute will be sufficient. If you buy reflexology sandals then only wear them for a few minutes a day, otherwise the reflexes will be over-worked.
2. Drink several glasses of water after a treatment to flush the wastes out of your system.
3. It is a good idea to rest after massaging your reflexology points so that the body can efficiently eliminate the toxins.
4. Never use reflexology in the first three months of pregnancy, after a heavy meal, or if you have been drinking alcohol. It is not advisable to use reflexology if you are suffering from deep vein thrombosis, diabetes, epilepsy, scar tissue or wounds, varicose veins or other serious illnesses. Please consult a qualified reflexologist if in doubt.

Acupressure

What Is Acupressure?

The system of acupressure is over 3,000 years old and has always been used in China, along with acupuncture, as a way of keeping the body healthy and strong. The Chinese discovered that when pressing specific points on the body for pain relief, this had a beneficial effect on other parts of the body that were not necessarily connected to the points being treated. These points, known as acupuncture points, are located on specific meridians (energy channels) running through the body. The points are named and numbered according to the specific meridian on which they are located.

How It Works

Acupressure is used for pain relief and as an all-round body balancing therapy that can not only release stress and tension held in the body, but support all the body organs and systems. It is therefore an excellent preventative technique. On a very simple level, tension and 'stagnation' (as the Chinese call it) can accumulate around certain acupoints, and this can cause physical symptoms such as muscle stiffness and fatigue. These are due to poor circulation, the build-up of chemicals such as lactic acid in the muscle fibres, and the disruption of the flow of *qi* around the body. Acupressure relaxes the muscles, so improving blood and oxygen supply locally to affected areas, and encouraging the smooth flow of *qi* once again.

Techniques

The Chinese use 'anatomical landmarks' such as the bones, and have a measurement known as a 'cun' to locate the points. In Western terms, 1 cun relates to the width of a finger, so elsewhere in this book I have used the term 'one finger width' to help you to locate the right acupoint.

When you have found the specific point, pressure is generally applied by using the pad of your thumb, or fingertip if you prefer. Keep your pressure on the points relatively light to start with, especially if you are sensitive or your body is fatigued and weak. The principle of 'no pain, no gain' does not apply here, rather wait until your energy and strength have improved and your body can naturally take more pressure. The point can be held for up to a minute or, alternatively, pressure can be applied intermittently by pressing on the point and then releasing the pressure. Small circular massage movements can also be applied to acupressure points. As acupressure points are bilateral (on both sides of the body), do remember to treat the related point on the other side of the body.

The length of time that the point is held will vary from individual to individual depending on his or her sensitivity and whether the problem is acute. In general, the principle of 'little and often' can be applied, with specific points being massaged or held for up to a minute at a time. If there is extreme pain or discomfort, acupressure can be carried out every two hours until there is improvement. For chronic conditions, acupressure should be done several times a week and continued over a few months for the best results.

General guidelines

1. Never use acupressure if you have consumed too much alcohol, are on strong drugs, or after a heavy meal.
2. Never use a specific pressure point if there is a wart, scar or wound on it.
3. If you suffer from heart trouble or any other serious illness, consult your GP or a trained practitioner before undertaking this type of treatment.
4. Avoid acupressure in the early or very late stages of pregnancy.
5. Never overstimulate a point or be too heavy-handed with the pressure on a point. Holding a point strengthens the energy for symptoms of deficiency; rubbing it can sedate excessive energy.
6. Drink several glasses of water (preferably warm!) after a treatment, to help flush waste out of your system.
7. Rest after massaging your points so that your body can efficiently eliminate toxins.

Aromatherapy

What Is Aromatherapy?

Aromatherapy is the use of aromatic essential oils from flowers, trees, fruits and herbs which help to heal the body on all levels (mind, body and spirit). It has a very strong impact on the whole person and can be classified as a 'holistic' therapy.

It is certainly not a new therapy, although it has become very popular over the last few decades. In fact, Hippocrates once said that *'the way to health is to have an aromatic bath and scented massage every day'*. The Egyptians in 4500 BC used the oils in many ways, and ointments containing frankincense and spikenard have recently been found in the tomb of Tutankhamen. In 2000 BC, the Emperor of China wrote about his discoveries regarding the properties of specific plants. Using herbs and oils for healing purposes (along with acupuncture) represents part of the unbroken Chinese tradition which remains to this day. In this century, a French chemist named René-Maurice Gattefossé burned his hand accidentally while working in his laboratory. He plunged his arm into a vat of Lavender oil and his burn not only healed quickly, but there was no infection and no scar. He dedicated the rest of his life to researching the amazing beneficial properties of plants and flowers. He wrote a book on the subject called *Aromathérapie*, thus giving this healing system a name it has kept ever since.

How It Works

Oils have many properties. They can be calming and sedative, analgesic, detoxifying, antiviral and antibacterial; others are revitalizing and stimulating, and even possess aphrodisiac properties. Certain oils and herbs also have an affinity for different organs in the body. For example, garlic goes to the lungs – if you rub a clove of garlic on the soles of your feet, 15 minutes later your breath will smell of garlic!

- Oils can penetrate the skin, and as Gattefossé first discovered, extra-cellular liquids take the oils into the circulatory and lymphatic systems. The oils tend to be carried into the body through the skin via a massage treatment.
- Aromatherapy oils are diluted in a carrier oil such as almond, grapeseed or sunflower, then massaged into the skin. As a general guide, 1 drop of essential oil should be mixed with 5 ml of carrier oil. **Check whether the essential oil is classified as weak, medium or strong; if the essential oil is weak, add 2 drops to 5 ml of oil; if medium, add 1 drop to 10 ml of oil; if strong, add 1 drop to 20 – 30 ml of oil.**
- Aromatherapy oils added to the bath are another wonderful way to enjoy aromatherapy; add a maximum of 8 drops as a rule. Use less if the oil is medium or strong (this information is listed with each oil later in the book).
- Smell is another powerful way in which we can absorb essential oils. The oils enter the lungs and can affect on our nervous system, hormones, emotions and moods. I often fill a spray bottle with water and add a few refreshing oils to stimulate my grey matter while I am researching and writing.
- Steam inhalations are excellent for colds and sinus infections. Add 2 to 3 drops of your chosen essential oil into a bowl of hot water, place your head above the bowl and drape a towel over. Breathe in the vapours, coming up for air when necessary!
- Oil burners are also readily available today, but do choose one

with an ample sized water dish. Otherwise, the water evaporates so quickly that your mixture burns in the water dish, and this leaves a far from pleasant smell! Approximately 5 drops can be added, depending on the size of the dish.

General guidelines

1. Certain oils are toxic in concentrated dosages, so if your knowledge of oils is limited, consult a professional aromatherapist who can advise you on what oils would be suitable and in what dosage.
2. The strength of each oil is classified as strong, medium or weak.
3. If using oils in the bath, add them when you have filled the bath, *do not mix them with the hot water directly from the tap*. Keep the bathroom door closed so that the vapours don't escape. Ensure that you relax in the bath for at least seven minutes before using any soap or shampoo, to get the maximum benefit from the oil.
4. When using citrus oils, it is advisable to mix them in a carrier oil before adding them to your bath water. If you were to add them neat and the drops did not disperse properly, they could burn your skin.
5. Keep oils away from your eyes as they can sting.
6. Purchase the very best oils that you can afford (preferably organic), and ensure that they are both pure and natural, as synthetic versions are now available which do not have the potency and effectiveness of true, unadulterated essential oils.
7. Do not have an aromatherapy treatment if you have consumed alcohol, are on drugs, or after a heavy meal.
8. Do not have an aromatherapy massage if you have a high fever or an illness such as influenza. If you suffer from any other serious illness, consult your GP or a trained aromatherapist before treatment.
9. Avoid aromatherapy in the early or very late stages of pregnancy and avoid using Marjoram, Fennel, Ginger, Peppermint and Rosemary oils at these times. Aromatherapy is beneficial during other stages of pregnancy, although it is best not to massage the abdomen.

10. If you suffer from epilepsy, avoid Fennel and Rosemary oils, and consult your doctor before you begin any treatment.
11. Strong oils such as Peppermint, Camphor, Black Pepper and Eucalyptus can counteract homoeopathic remedies, so do speak to a qualified homoeopath if you are using both therapies.
12. Drink several glasses of water after an aromatherapy treatment to flush the wastes out of your system. It is also a good idea to rest after a massage so that the body can efficiently eliminate toxins and regenerate body tissues.

The Emotions

Today, Western medicine is at long last beginning to validate the healing power not only of the body, but of the mind. Exciting research has transformed our concept of the mind and it is now thought that the mind has a presence throughout the entire body. This is because the cells which carry emotions in the brain have recently been discovered to exist in our immune system. The Chinese have understood for thousands of years that our thoughts and emotions have a great impact on the state of our health and that emotional distress compromises the health of the body. This is why emotions play an important role in this book and are discussed in each of the chapters on the organs. There are five emotions, which are connected to the five elements and to the major *yin* organs (the liver, heart, spleen, lungs and kidneys). Anger relates to the liver, joy to the heart, pensiveness to the spleen, grief to the lungs and fear to the kidneys.

Flower Remedies

What Are Flower Remedies?
Flower essences are liquids that have been infused with individual plants and flowers. They have the capacity to restore wellbeing to the body on all levels, the physical, mental, emotional and spiritual. It is believed that flowers possess special healing powers due to their energetic and vibrational qualities and that every type of flower has a totally unique energy system and characteristics.

The traditional way of making a flower essence is to put the petals of the flower in a bowl of water and leave them in the sun for several hours to allow the flowers to 'infuse'. This tincture is diluted and preserved with an alcohol such as brandy. Several drops of the resulting remedy are taken on a daily basis.

Flower essences have been used for thousands of years in many different countries. For example, the Native Americans used to match the energies of specific flowers to particular parts of the body that needed healing. In England, Dr Bach, a one-time successful London doctor who became disillusioned with ortho-dox medical practice, devoted his life after leaving the medical profession to researching the healing power and energy of plants. He eventually isolated 38 different flowers to help heal specific emotional upsets: the Bach flower remedies were born. I have included these remedies in this book as they are easily available in Europe and other parts of the world.

How They Work

Unlike conventional drug therapies, which work primarily on the physical level, the energetic patterns contained within flower essences work best on the emotional, spiritual and mental levels. Flower remedies work in a similar way to homoeopathic remedies in as much as they are a form of subtle energy. The vibrational energy of the plant is captured in the remedy and, when taken orally, helps bring us into a state of harmony by dissolving blockages on the emotional and mental levels (such as worry, fear, anxiety). Once we are in balance again, the state of disease subsides.

General guidelines

1. Bach flower remedies have no side-effects, are not habit-forming, and can be used safely on both adults and children.
2. For a single remedy, 4 drops are taken in water. The same is true of Rescue remedy, the classic composite Bach flower remedy for shock and trauma.
3. You can take more than one remedy at a time, although some practitioners advocate that you take no more than four different remedies in a specific mixture. If you decide to take several remedies together, take approximately 2 drops of each in a glass of water, or neat under the tongue.

Affirmations

Affirmations are short, positive statements which you repeat out aloud or silently to yourself to help in the process of change. They can help us to achieve many things including better health and higher levels of self-esteem and self-worth. In the early stages of working with affirmations, one of the most important things that they can do is to help counterbalance negative, self-defeating messages that play in our head. We all suffer from this inner dialogue, fears and worries about our health, our abilities, relationships, self-worth, etc. These worries can be greatly reduced by controlling the way we think. If we gradually replace negative statements with an affirmation that is supportive and nourishing, this will help retrain and reprogramme the subconscious mind to think in a more positive and constructive way.

Don't panic if at first you find it difficult, just remember that you will be challenging beliefs which you have most probably been carrying since your early years of life! Put effort and passion into them, as saying affirmations mechanically without having any belief or expectations about them will certainly not carry as much power as those said with feeling.

The affirmations in this book are tailored specifically to the organ systems and to reinforcing the emotions that relate to the various organs. You can have great fun making up affirmations, so don't hesitate in trying to formulate your own unique statements. Just keep them positive and easy to say. They can be as simple as *I am healthy* or *I feel wonderful* or *I like myself* (better still, *I love myself*!).

Smiling has been proved to boost the immune system and improve health. The physiological changes in the facial muscles are enough to stimulate endorphins, our 'happy pills' from the pharmacy in our head. So try smiling while you say your affirmations; this will boost your mood even more!

Visualization and Meditation

There is much research both to support and prove the power of visualization and meditation in overcoming disease and bringing the body back to a state of equilibrium. Visualizations are a way of using the power of our imagination to build constructive, supportive images which help to replace deep-seated negative conditioning and attract a new level of health and well-being. They can be used to enhance any area of your life, but the chapters on individual organs focus on visualizations designed to balance and positively transform specific body systems, to enhance and build your general health.

When you try some of the meditations outlined in this book, do not be concerned if you cannot 'see' images. We are all different and some of us can feel, some of us sense – just use whatever process works best for you.

It is advisable to tape the meditations so that you can fully relax, or have a friend read them to you. Remember to speak *very* slowly and in a gentle and relaxed manner.

What Element are You?
– Questionnaire

This questionnaire is designed to help you find out whether you have a main element (Earth, Fire, Water, Wood or Metal) that is out of balance and needs support. When answering the questionnaire, be as honest as possible and do not reflect for too long over the question, as the most immediate response is normally the most accurate.

Scoring System

- If you suffer from these symptoms very frequently, or you resonate strongly with the emotional picture, score: **3**
- If you suffer from these symptoms and emotions regularly, score: **1**
- If you suffer from these symptoms and emotions occasionally, score: **0**
- If you only have these problems once in a while, or feel indifferent towards the question, score: **-1**
- If you have a strong negative response as you never experience these emotions or symptoms, score: **-3**

Earth Element – Stomach and Spleen

1. Abdominal distension and bloating ☐
2. Puffiness, water retention and mucus in the body ☐
3. Tired, aching, heavy and cold limbs ☐
4. Great fatigue and lethargy ☐
5. Flabby, weak flesh, lack of muscle tone and strength in lower body ☐
6. Prolapsed organs in lower body, bladder, intestines, uterus ☐
7. Loose stools and diarrhoea, abdominal gas and flatulence ☐
8. Poor digestion and assimilation of food, slow metabolism ☐
9. Pain under the left side of the rib cage near the spleen and stomach ☐
10. Symptoms are aggravated by cold, damp and humid conditions ☐
11. Easily worried and over-concerned ☐
12. Obsessional and compulsive behaviour disorder ☐
13. Upset by change and tendency to become overwhelmed by detail ☐
14. Eating disorders such as bulimia and anorexia nervosa ☐
15. Craving for sweet foods and ice-cream ☐
16. Worse from eating cold foods, sweets and raw fruit and vegetables ☐
17. Appetite imbalance, either voracious or lack of appetite ☐
18. Hiccups and burping, nausea and vomiting ☐
19. Worse between the hours of 7 and 11 a.m. ☐
20. Acid in the stomach, duodenal or gastric ulcers ☐

TOTAL ☐

Fire Element – Heart and Small Intestine

1. Palpitations and panic attacks ☐
2. Heart attacks, angina, hardening of the arteries ☐
3. High or very low blood pressure ☐
4. Poor circulation ☐
5. Fatigue with restlessness and anxiety ☐
6. Insomnia and hot flushes in the night ☐
7. Highly coloured complexion ☐

8. Vivid dreams, restless sleep and nightmares ☐
9. Extreme anxiety, emotional unease and lack of joy ☐
10. Hatred and cruel behaviour ☐
11. Lack of self-love and low self-worth ☐
12. Excessive laughter and giggling at inappropriate times ☐
13. Poor muscle tone and swollen abdomen ☐
14. Pain in the throat, shoulder and neck ☐
15. Tennis elbow and frozen shoulder ☐
16. Symptoms are aggravated by excess heat ☐
17. Mental confusion and indecision ☐
18. Unable to make decisions ☐
19. Worse between the hours of 11 a.m. and 3 p.m. ☐
20. Hearing difficulties and deafness ☐

TOTAL ☐

Water Element – Bladder and Kidneys

1. Poor bladder control, frequent urination ☐
2. Cystitis and bladder infections ☐
3. Puffiness and water retention around the ankles and feet ☐
4. Puffiness and dark bags under the eyes ☐
5. Infertility and impotence ☐
6. Low libido and lack of sexual fluids ☐
7. Constant tiredness, lethargy and frequent yawning ☐
8. Pain in the lower back, sciatica and lumbago ☐
9. Stiffness or weakness of the knees ☐
10. Tightness or soreness in the back of the legs and hips ☐
11. Pain in arches, soles and heels of feet ☐
12. Thin hair, split ends, lack of shine ☐
13. Premature greying of hair, loss of hair ☐
14. Symptoms are aggravated by cold and damp conditions ☐
15. Fears and phobias; timidity and lack of confidence ☐
16. Paranoid and suspicious behaviour ☐
17. Constant complaining and moaning ☐
18. Craving for salty foods ☐

19. Soft or brittle, weak bones ☐
20. Learning difficulties, slow development, poor memory recall ☐

TOTAL ☐

Wood Element – Gallbladder and Liver

1. Nauseous headaches and migraines ☐
2. Premenstrual symptoms including mood changes and breast tenderness ☐
3. Irregular and painful periods, inflamed genital organs ☐
4. Weak eyesight, sore, tired, dry eyes and spots in front of eyes (floaters) ☐
5. Weak, ridged and splitting nails ☐
6. Stiffness and rigidity in the muscles, especially in the shoulders and neck ☐
7. Problems with tendons and ligaments, lack of flexibility ☐
8. Dizziness and nausea, vomiting brought on by food avoidance ☐
9. Shouting and a loud voice ☐
10. Pain under the right side of the ribcage near the liver and gallbladder ☐
11. Difficulty digesting fatty foods, allergies and low tolerance to alcohol ☐
12. Bitter or metallic taste in the mouth ☐
13. Symptoms are aggravated by wind and draughts ☐
14. Poor organizational and planning skills ☐
15. Frustration, anger, aggression, irritability and extreme nervous tension ☐
16. Jealousy and resentment, unexpressed anger leading to depression ☐
17. Twitches and spasms in the body and muscles ☐
18. Craving for sour foods such as pickles and lemons ☐
19. Worse between the hours of 11 p.m. and 3 a.m. ☐
20. Clumsy and accident prone ☐

TOTAL ☐

Metal Element – Lungs and Large Intestine

1. Breathing difficulties, asthma, emphysema ☐
2. Shortness of breath and fatigue on exertion ☐
3. Tightness in the chest and a soft voice ☐
4. Frequent cold and infections, low immunity ☐
5. Coughing with or without phlegm, throat infections, laryngitis ☐
6. Sinusitis, sneezing, rhinitis and other nasal difficulties ☐
7. Excess mucus or, alternatively, dryness and lack of mucus ☐
8. Excessive or lack of perspiration ☐
9. Poor sense of smell ☐
10. Constipation and diarrhoea ☐
11. Strong smelly odours from faeces or flatulence ☐
12. Body odour and bad breath ☐
13. Pain in the chest or in the lower abdomen ☐
14. Aggravated by heat and dryness ☐
15. Dryness of the skin, psoriasis and eczema ☐
16. Grief, pessimism, melancholy, weeping and depression ☐
17. Unable to 'let go' of the past, bored and apathetic behaviour ☐
18. Craving for spicy and pungent foods ☐
19. Worse between the hours of 3 and 7 a.m. ☐
20. Poor memory and fuzzy thinking ☐

TOTAL ☐

The Results

Add your scores up for each element: you should have a higher score for one. You can now turn to the relevant chapter to understand more about the organ(s) and what you can do to help yourself.

Due to the nature of the organs and their interrelationships, we can sometimes have several elements producing symptoms. If a clear picture does not emerge after completing the questionnaire, refer to the chapters on the individual organs and see which element(s) are most applicable to you.

PART III

The Earth Element

Partner Organs: The spleen is paired with the stomach and assists in the 'transformation and transportation' of food and drink. The action of chewing prepares the food for the transforming and transporting work of the stomach and spleen. If food is not properly transformed by either organ, this can lead to a build-up of excessive dampness (water retention and mucus), and congestion. This saps our vitality and further weakens digestion, giving rise to symptoms such as fullness and bloating, lack of appetite, hiccups, loose stools and flatulence, and contributes towards a sluggish lymphatic system.

Climate: The climate for the Earth element is humidity and dampness, both of which can weaken the functions of the stomach and spleen. If your symptoms are aggravated by either type of climate, this is a diagnostic clue to where your imbalances lie.

Season: The Earth phase is associated with Late Summer – or Indian Summer, as it is often known. It is a time of balance, transformation and neutrality. Describing it in nature's cycles, the Earth phase is when the flowers from Summer have transformed themselves into fruits. It is a time of ripening, just like the key function of one of the Earth organs, the stomach, 'ripening and rotting'. It encompasses everything about the Earth and exemplifies being steady, grounded and secure, with the fruits of the harvest in abundance.

Colour: Yellow is the colour associated with the Earth element and is reflected in the golden hues that are so prevalent in Late Summer. When there is a spleen imbalance, a TCM practitioner with a trained eye will be able to detect a yellow tinge in skin tone. A passion for the colour or, conversely, a strong dislike of yellow, can point to an imbalance in this element.

Time of Day: 7 to 9 a.m. (stomach) and 9 to 11 a.m. (spleen) – good times for the stomach to begin digesting food and for the spleen to finish this 'transformation'.

Body Tissue: The spleen controls the condition of our flesh and muscles; a firm, toned body is a good indication of strong spleen energy. On the other hand, poor circulation, obesity, flabby flesh, lack of muscle tone, feelings of fatigue or heaviness in the legs, weak muscles and atrophy of the flesh also connect to the Earth element. Then the texture of the flesh is not smooth; it has the appearance of a watery version of cellulite. Poor circulation is more common in women; one reason this is thought to be so is that menstruation is dependent on strong spleen energy and a monthly loss of blood puts a strain on this organ as it has to generate more blood to replace this.

Voice Sound: Speaking with a melodic tone points to the spleen and stomach, as a singing sound relates to these organs.

Sense Organ: The mouth is the orifice or opening governed by the Earth element and has a direct relationship with the spleen. The mouth secretes saliva, which is the fluid secretion of the Earth element; a deficiency of this will prevent food from being digested properly.

Reflector: The lips are thought to reflect the strength of the stomach and spleen. When they are moist and rosy, these organs are healthy and strong; when they are pale and dry, these organs need some attention.

Symptoms of Imbalance: Obsessions, worry, poor memory, excessive dampness of the body (water retention, excessive mucus), weight gain, congested lymphatic system, prolapse and loose stools.

The Stomach

 The stomach is a flexible J-shaped sac located on the left-hand side of the body, just beneath the diaphragm. It has the dual function of receiving and digesting foods.

Western Function

Digestion begins in the mouth where saliva starts to break down the starches in food into simple forms of sugar. The saliva moistens the food and makes it pass down more easily through a tube called the oesophagus which leads into the stomach. Powerful acidic digestive juices are released in the stomach to help break down proteins. The contraction and relaxation of the muscles of the stomach wall help to mix the food with enzymes, turning it into a liquid called chyme. This partially digested food is then released into a tube called the duodenum, which is where the gallbladder and pancreas secrete more juices to continue the process of digestion.

Traditional Chinese Interpretation

Element:	Earth
Partner organ:	Spleen
Climate:	Humidity
Season:	Late Summer
Colour:	Yellow
Time of day:	7–9 a.m.
Body tissue:	Muscles/flesh
Voice sound:	Singing
Sense organ:	Mouth
Reflector:	Lips
Taste:	Sweet
Emotion:	Sympathy/worry

SYMPTOMS OF IMBALANCE

Emotional
Emotional worries that constantly gnaw away inside your
stomach •• Insecurity • Craving sympathy

Physical
Duodenal and gastric ulcers • Chronic gastritis • Poor or
voracious appetite • Nausea, vomiting • Hiccups • Belching •
Colic • Dyspepsia (pain in digestive tract)

In TCM the stomach is called the 'Sea of Nourishment' and is the
first part of 'receiving and transforming' food and drink into energy.
The stomach 'rots and ripens the food', sends the impure to the
small intestine and the pure up to the spleen, where the resultant
energy is distributed. When this works efficiently, digestion and
metabolism are perfect and the appetite strong. This is the why
some people can get away with eating large quantities of food
without gaining weight. Conversely, someone with a weak stomach
and digestion can put on 3 kg just by looking at a cream cake!

The stomach energy is downward, so water and nutrients
should naturally move downwards, allowing the process of

digestion, assimilation and excretion to take place. If the energy is disturbed and moves in an upward direction, symptoms such as belching, hiccups, nausea and vomiting will arise.

SELF-HELP FOR KEEPING YOUR STOMACH HEALTHY

Chinese Nutrition

Foods for the Earth Element

Grain: millet	Fruit: apricot
Meat: beef (organic)	Vegetable: scallions

The food that we consume is a major contributing factor to the health and wellbeing of the stomach. Equally, our approach to eating food is significant. Traditionally, the Chinese stress the importance of eating meals at regular times, something which is very alien to many people today. Often we eat a meal or snack for the sake of it instead of allowing the body to produce enough hydrochloric acid to digest the food consumed efficiently. Without real hunger, the food that goes into the stomach will not be properly broken down and this will, at some point, create problems.

A simple way of knowing if your body has produced this acid and is ready to digest a meal is to experience and awaken the hungry dragon within who should be bellowing 'feed me'. That hungry feeling before a meal, when you can't wait any longer to be fed, is your body's way of demonstrating that the digestive juices are ready to break down food into smaller particles. Very often we eat when the body is not really ready to digest food. We may be stressed or have just had a row and then sit down to a meal. The body cannot digest food efficiently under these circumstances.

Experience has shown that irregular eating habits go on to produce stomach disorders. The following advice is, therefore, as important as the food you eat:

Dietary Tips

1. Do not over-eat, as this prevents the stomach from digesting food properly.
2. Constant nibbling and eating too fast does not give the stomach enough time to digest the food.
3. Eating late at night causes the body to use its *yin* energy (as night is the time for *yin*), putting a strain on the digestive system. It doesn't like to start the process all over again at night!
4. Under-eating or malnourishment due to strict diets lacking in basic nourishment can weaken the stomach and spleen energy.
5. Eating on the run or while standing up is not advised as it can cause the stagnation of stomach energy.
6. Eating when worried or stressed, no matter how pure and wholesome the food may be, will not do any good and, like eating on the run, can contribute to burning pains, belching and nausea. Eating when angry also has an indirect action via the liver and can cause abdominal distension and pain.

NB A good home remedy if you do suffer from indigestion is to mix a tablespoon of 'live' natural yoghurt containing lactobacillus acidophilus into a glass of water and drink it – this should quickly soothe and remove any irritating pains in the stomach region. Peppermint, chamomile and ginger herbal teas can also help to ease indigestion.

If you suffer from digestive fermentation and bloating, food combining may be a useful regime to try. This is where you do not eat concentrated starches and concentrated proteins at the same time. There are many books on the market that go into greater detail and also include tasty recipes (*see Further Reading, page 217*). For a short cut, another idea is to 'food stack'. This means that you eat the protein part of your meal first so that the concentrated hydrochloric acid juices in the stomach can break the food down more efficiently. Follow this with the starches; so eat the meat or fish followed by carbohydrates such as rice or potato. Remember to chew your food well, as the starches are first broken down in the mouth; this practice alone will help strengthen weak digestion greatly. Keep your intake of sugar, yeast and alcohol low, as this can increase fermentation and bloating. When digestion is poor, eat nuts only in moderation, as they can put a strain on the system, especially if it is weak to begin with, and restrict your intake of fatty foods such as butter and mayonnaise.

If you suffer from diarrhoea, hiccups and abdominal pains, try eating the following foods:

- star anise, cayenne pepper (in small quantities), fresh ginger, black and white pepper, cloves, chestnuts, ham, garlic, pistachio nut, beef and dates.
- Yellow mustard, fennel, nutmeg and cinnamon can be added to the list if there is fatigue, chilliness and a pale complexion.

If you have stomach ulcers:

- Avoid spicy foods, alcohol, and herbs such as black pepper, chillies, etc. as they can create too much heat in the stomach.
- Cabbage and cabbage juice have long been used to cure stomach and duodenal ulcers – the active ingredient being vitamin U. Fennel, lettuce and potato juice are also helpful.

Foods that strengthen the stomach and Earth element:

- Millet is the grain for the spleen and is one of the oldest cultivated grains known to man. It contains seven of the eight essential amino acids and is said to help improve your physical appearance as well as create emotional balance.
- Sweet potatoes, yams and squashes, root vegetables and tubers support the spleen and stomach and are in season in Late Summer, the Earth time in Chinese medicine.
- Parsnips are pale yellow and when baked in the oven (and caramelized) have a wonderful sweet taste, the taste associated with the Earth element. They are high in vitamin A, potassium and calcium.
- Sweet potatoes are thought to warm the stomach, strengthen the internal organs and support body energy. They are rich in carbohydrates, beta carotene (which is converted to vitamin A in the liver) and potassium.
- Yellow squash is high in all the life-giving minerals and vitamins including vitamin A, calcium, potassium, magnesium and phosphorus.

Other strengthening foods for the Earth element include apricots, apples (all fruit preferably lightly stewed), chickpeas, cherries, courgettes, cucumbers, dates, grapes, lamb, lettuce, mung beans, oats, peaches, pears, plums, pork, potatoes, raspberries, rice, spinach, strawberries and walnuts.

Helpful herbs and spices
- Ginger tea is excellent for strengthening digestion and relieving nausea. Make a cup by boiling dried root ginger for 20 minutes. Drink this tea 30 minutes prior to every meal; over time, your digestion will be strengthened.
- If there is heat or inflammation in the stomach, peppermint tea can soothe the area and also help to alleviate indigestion.
- Fennel herb tea can also help with indigestion or trapped wind in the digestive tract.
- Bland herbs such as slippery elm and marshmallow can soothe and calm an irritated stomach. Slippery elm can coat the inside of the stomach, allowing tissue healing and regeneration to take place.
- Liquorice promotes the healing of the mucus membranes lining the stomach wall. Two derivatives of liquorice root can reduce the size of an ulcer by 70 – 90 per cent after one month of treatment.
- Digestive bitter herbs, which can be purchased from good health food shops, also aid digestion.

Exercise

Some form of movement is essential for the Earth element, as over-work and excess sitting is thought to weaken the stomach and spleen meridians. However, if there is muscle weakness you probably won't have the stamina for a great deal. Therefore, start gradually by doing 15–20 minutes of gentle exercise every day. Walking in the fresh air and breathing deeply would be a very good start. As your muscles get stronger, you can increase both the duration and intensity of the exercise, but never over-exert yourself.

The stretch for the spleen and stomach meridian begins by adopting a kneeling position and placing your hands on the floor. Keeping the spine straight, slowly inhale and put the weight on your hands. Exhale and push your hips towards the ceiling, dropping your head back and trying to relax into the position. Feel the stretch running down the front of your thighs and torso. Remember that it may take many weeks or months to achieve this. Always work at your own pace and ensure that you have warmed the muscles in your body for 10 minutes prior to stretching. If possible, join a local yoga class where you can be guided and personally instructed.

The stomach/spleen stretch

Reflexology points for the stomach (shaded)

Touch Therapies

Reflexology

Massage the reflex points for the stomach, found mostly on the inner side of the left foot. The same area on the right foot can also be massaged. (*See page 30 for massage techniques.*)

Acupressure

The stomach meridian begins just below the eye then runs to the jawbone and, after reaching the collarbone, travels inside and so connects with the stomach internally. It resurfaces near the pubic

The stomach meridian

Stomach 36 acupressure point

bone and descends down the front of the thigh and along to finish at the base of the nail on the second toe, next to the big toe.

STOMACH 36

The main energizing point on this meridian is located 5 cm beneath the outer part of the knee bone, just on the outside of the shin. This powerful point helps to fight fatigue and support the whole body. It also helps with indigestion and can give relief to other disorders of the stomach, as well as strengthening the whole digestive system. If combined with its partner organ's key point, Spleen 6, the effect will be even stronger (*see Figure, page 71*). When pressing this point, visualize a brilliant golden sun-shine colour in and around the point and say the spleen sound, 'WHOOOOOO'.

This is a superb point to burn a moxa stick over (*see Part I for details on moxibustion*), which helps strengthen weak digestion and improve energy levels.

Essential Oils

Caraway: promotes circulation in the digestive system and has a calming action on the stomach. Helpful for indigestion, pain, belching and bloating. *Strength factor: Strong*

Cardamom: for digestive disorders which are caused by nervous strain and worry. Settles feelings of nausea and treats colic, hiccoughs, indigestion, poor appetite, trapped wind and abdominal bloating. Also a mild brain tonic.
Strength factor: Strong

Coriander: has a warming and drying action which helps to circulate the energy in the stomach and lower digestive tract. Fortifies weak individuals suffering from exhaustion and is useful for nervous depression caused by excessive worry.
Strength factor: Strong

Fennel: Regulates appetite. Fennel tea (as well as the oil being massaged on to the abdomen) has a tonic effect on both the stomach and intestine and can relieve colic, indigestion, nausea, hiccoughs and trapped gas. *Strength factor: Strong*

Ginger: for painful digestion, abdominal distension, loss of appetite, travel sickness (and morning sickness), hangovers and nausea. On an emotional level, it is good for the Earth personality who is over-dependent on others and over-whelmed by self-doubt. *Strength factor: Medium*

Peppermint: for acute symptoms such as abdominal pain, indigestion, vomiting, diarrhoea. A very weak dilution of peppermint oil can be applied to the stomach area (less than 1 per cent dilution – 1 drop maximum mixed with 30 ml carrier oil). Drinking peppermint tea helps as well. Also helps with flatulence, food poisoning, travel sickness (keep peppermints in your car for emergencies!). Relaxes and sedates the stomach muscles. Mentally stimulating as well. *Strength factor: Strong*

Emotions

Food can spend many hours being processed, and emotions can ferment too, creating nausea and tension. A rigid stomach can indicate a resistance to allowing issues to pass through, be digested and finally released. Look at a classic example of how when you are *worried* about an event, your stomach gets tied up in knots and you feel nauseous and sick. If this worry and anxiety is never addressed, but continues to 'gnaw away inside you', the outcome on a physical level could be that the body produces an ulcer.

One simple, cheap and highly effective preventative tool is laughter. Researchers have found that those who laugh frequently are less prone to ulcers and other digestive disturbances. Laughter can stabilize and improve many bodily functions and encourage tissue healing.

There are so many emotive issues that surround food, and advertisers are well aware of this. They use it to its full advantage, seducing us into eating food that titillates our palate but does nothing for our long-term health and vitality. We have a real problem with caring for ourselves and taking the necessary time to feel that we are important enough to nourish ourselves with both enjoyable and nutritional food.

Issues of self-nourishment are often tied up with eating disorders. Food represents mother, lover, affection, security, survival and reward. We often replace our need or desire for any one of these with food as a way of filling the emptiness within. Food is used as a substitute for affection and love, especially during stressful times. Eating excess sweet food (the taste of the Earth element being sweet) is a way of giving ourselves the sweetness or reward that we may feel nobody else is giving to us. Conversely, starvation regimes express the state of not wanting to nourish or care for ourselves.

The path to breaking some of these addictive patterns is to recognize that there is a problem. The next stage is to make a conscious decision to talk about it to a friend or counsellor, rather than bottling it up. Also, make sure that you then get involved in some form of constructive activity to replace the habit of over-eating or not eating enough. Look at the issues surrounding your lack of self-worth and ways that you can build on this and im-prove your self-confidence.

Flower Remedies

Chicory: the remedy for 'mothering' types who constantly worry. This love can sometimes turn into possessive and demanding behaviour. Helps to develop the gift of unconditional love.

White Chestnut: for times when your mind just will not switch off and your thoughts constantly churn. The remedy can encourage you to get into the habit of assessing problems objectively and talking about your feelings, then deciding on the appropriate course of action to help bring solutions to your problems.

Affirmations

- My stomach digests food calmly and efficiently.
- I understand that nourishing my body on all levels is essential and that I am worthy of receiving this nourishment.
- I trust my stomach to break down the food which I lovingly eat.
- I am centred and feel satisfied with my life.

See also the Spleen chapter, page 65, for affirmations that may be used in conjunction with these.

Meditation for the Earth Element

Before beginning this meditation, familiarize yourself with the diagrams of the relevant meridians (i.e. for the stomach and spleen). Remember that *qi* is pronounced 'chee', and that all meridians are bilateral (running along both sides of the body); for the purposes of this meditation, focus on the meridian points on only one side of the body. If possible, tape the meditation, reading it out clearly and slowly in a soft tone of voice.

Find a peaceful place to relax and unwind. Close your eyes. Focus your attention on your breathing and, as you begin to notice it deepening, gently let any thoughts that come into your mind float by like clouds in the sky. For a few minutes, practise the breathing exercise recommended in the Lung chapter (*page 183*).

Earth Meditation

Imagine yourself lying amongst fruit trees in an orchard on a warm and mellow day in late Summer. The trees are heavily laden with ripened fruit: golden juicy pears, rosy red apples and sweet succulent plums. As you look at all that Nature has to offer at this abundant time of year, feel a sense of appreciation for the rich gifts that this harvest brings. Feel an empathy with the warm earth, supporting and nurturing you.

Now imagine that with every out-breath, a root grows from the base of your spine and smaller roots spread from the end of your toes, going deep into the centre of the earth. As you inhale, feel your body absorbing energy from Mother Earth. Visualize this energy as a golden liquid and see it filling your entire body, right up to the top of your head.

Now focus this energy just below your left eye, the start of the Stomach meridian. Feel it flow over the front of your body, down the outside of your leg, until it reaches Stomach 36, located just below your knee. Hold and intensify the *qi* at this point, visualizing golden light penetrating and energizing this vital point, increasing the levels of *qi* in your body. When you feel that you have charged this point enough, feel the energy moving down your leg, finishing at your second toe. Now concentrate on the outside of your big toe just below the nail, where the Spleen meridian begins. Send the *qi* along your foot, until you reach Spleen 6, a point on the inside of your leg, then up the front of your body to the armpit region and back down to the spleen itself, and imagine this organ surrounded by golden light. Allow both your stomach and your spleen to absorb this healing light, enhancing and strengthening their ability to receive and transform Mother Earth's produce into vital energy for you.

Feel waves of golden energy washing over your whole body, filling your mind, body and spirit with a deep sense of satisfaction and fulfilment. Give thanks to Mother Earth. Sense your energy becoming stronger and begin to move your fingers and toes, feeling yourself revitalized and grounded ... and, in your own time, open your eyes and stretch your body out.

The Spleen

 The spleen is about half the size of your hand and is composed of soft tissue. It is situated under the left ribcage, just beneath the stomach. It is the largest organ of the lymphatic system.

Western Function

The main function of the spleen is to filter, store and clean blood. It destroys and eliminates any worn-out red blood cells and recycles them into iron for the production of haemoglobin and bile, which is taken to the liver. The spleen stores blood for emergency use; this is what gives the rich purple colour. It plays a key role in supporting the immune system, producing antibodies which help to neutralize and remove poisonous bacteria and foreign invaders.

The pancreas is located behind the stomach and is connected to the small intestine via a tube. It is part of the endocrine system and is about 15 cm long. It secretes enzymes which help break down the foods in the small intestine and is also involved in balancing blood sugar levels in the body. Pancreatic juice is the only one that digests all three kinds of food: proteins, fats and carbohydrates. The pancreas produces two hormones: insulin and glucagon. Glucagon converts glycogen stored in the liver into glucose (sugar) to raise blood sugar levels and provide an immediate source of energy for the body. Conversely, insulin lowers blood sugar levels by converting excess glucose into glycogen for storage in the liver or into fat to be stored away.

Traditional Chinese Interpretation

Element:	Earth
Partner organ:	Stomach
Climate:	Humidity
Season:	Late Summer
Colour:	Yellow
Time of day:	9–11 a.m.
Body tissue:	Muscles/flesh
Voice sound:	Singing
Sense organ:	Mouth
Reflector:	Lips
Taste:	Sweet
Emotion:	Sympathy/worry

SYMPTOMS OF IMBALANCE

Emotional
Feeling ungrounded and unearthed • Insecurity and instability • Worry and obsession • Restless sleep • Needy and selfish behaviour • Confusion and vagueness • Negative recurring thoughts • Poor concentration • Scattered feelings • Over-protective of others • 'Stuck' behaviour

---

Physical
Abdominal distension • Bloating and water retention • Prolapse
and sagging of the body • Tired body, heavy and aching limbs •
Poor co-ordination and dyslexic tendencies • Swollen, cold knees
and thighs • Loose stools and diarrhoea • Yellowish face and
body • Accumulations of dampness and mucus • Urinary
problems and vaginal discharge • Poor memory • Appetite
imbalance • Nourishment issues • Aversion to dampness

In Chinese medicine the pancreas has a very close link with the
spleen; the meridian is often referred to as the spleen/pancreas
meridian. The spleen's key role in TCM is to transform food, absorb
nourishment, extract *qi* and then separate the usable from the
unusable parts of food. The transformed food essences create the
basis for the formation of body energy or *qi* and blood, which is
then combined with the *qi* from the lungs, the two energies mixing
to form true energy which is distributed throughout the body.

The state of the spleen is one of the most important factors
determining the amount of physical energy a person has;
tiredness is a common complaint when this organ is weak. This is
because the spleen is the source of life for all other organs. It is in
charge of distribution, the transporter of energy. When not functioning efficiently, the body does not receive the energy it needs
on the physical, psychological and spiritual levels. The spleen is
known as the 'root of post-heaven *qi*', which means it is the
major source of all the energy which is produced by the body
after birth. As we shall see later, the kidney is the organ responsible for our 'pre-heaven' *qi*.

The spleen is the organ responsible for transforming food
essences into blood and governing the blood circulating
throughout the entire body. It ensures that the body is nourished
and is said to hold the blood securely in the blood vessels. The
spleen energy is also known to have a lifting effect on the body
and can hold organs in place, so disharmony in this organ can lead to
conditions such as internal prolapse, various types of bleeding
(including haemorrhages), chronic diarrhoea and tiredness.

SELF-HELP FOR KEEPING YOUR SPLEEN HEALTHY

Chinese Nutrition

Foods for the Earth Element

Grain: millet	Fruit: apricot
Meat: beef (organic)	Vegetable: scallions

The taste for this element is sweet, so if someone has an addiction for sweet foods, or a strong dislike of them, this can be a clue to look at the Earth element. We in the West tend to have an obsession with sweet food, but the excessive consumption of one type of food to the exclusion of others is not a sensible practice, as a variety of foods is necessary for our health and wellbeing.

The subject of food allergies is a huge topic in itself and is viewed in Chinese medicine as a symptom of poor digestion. It is important, therefore, to build the general health of the body and strengthen the spleen.

Raw food diets are very popular in the Western world, but in the East are not considered to be particularly beneficial. If you are cold or have a weak constitution, a raw food diet can exacerbate this state (please refer to the interior/exterior causes of disease, *page 10*). Some raw food in the diet does supply a rich supply of essential vitamins, minerals and vital enzymes, but long term, if these foods are over-used to the exclusion of other foods, they can deplete the 'digestive fire' (an Oriental term used to describe digestion). Too much cold and raw food will simply make the spleen go soggy and put the fire out, contributing to poor digestion.

It is important to understand that most things are fine in moderation, so if you enjoy juices and fruits, ensure that you also have some warm foods and spices in your diet to create *balance*. We are all individual and it is important to find out what creates balance and harmony for us personally. Keep an open mind and be prepared to adapt your diet to the seasons, climate and local produce available.

Dietary Tips

1. Reduce your consumption of raw foods and juices in the Autumn and Winter months.
2. As the spleen likes dryness, warm, dry foods are beneficial, as are warming spices such as cinnamon, nutmeg, ginger and cardamom, as well as ginseng, which is said to strengthen the spleen.
3. Millet is an alkaline, gluten-free grain which does not create mucus in the body. It can, however, be very stodgy if not prepared correctly. It must be soaked overnight and rinsed several times before cooking it for 10 minutes. This prevents it from becoming too sticky.
4. Sweet potatoes, yams and squashes, root vegetables such as parsnips, carrots and turnips support the spleen and are in season in Late Summer (Earth time).
5. Food recommendations to help drain dampness include aduki beans, alfalfa, barley, black pepper, cayenne pepper, celery, chicken, corn, dill seed, fennel, garlic, horseradish, kidney, kidney beans, lemon, lobster, mackerel, marjoram, mushrooms, mustard, mustard leaf, nutmeg, onion, parsley, pistachios, pumpkin, sardines and walnuts.
6. Other foods to strengthen the Earth element include apples, apricots, cherries, dates, grapes, peaches, pears, plums, raspberries, strawberries (all fruit preferably lightly stewed), chestnuts, chickpeas, courgettes, cucumbers, lamb, lettuce, mung beans, oats, peas, pork, potatoes, rice, spinach and string beans.
7. Black dates can help to replenish *qi* and relieve fatigue.
8. If there is a lot of water in the body, aduki beans, alfalfa, broad beans, celery, clams, fenugreek, lettuce, parsley and seaweed are the best foods to include in your diet.
9. If you include foods such as lettuce, it is worth having warm foods with it to help keep the spleen dry, or making a salad dressing with grated ginger to go over the lettuce.
10. Foods which have significant blood sugar-lowering action to support the pancreas are artichokes, Brussels sprouts, buckwheat, cucumber, garlic, green beans, oats, onions, soya beans and other legumes/pulses and spirulina.

11. Individuals with weak spleens need to ensure that they have adequate amounts of good quality protein in their diet, as this stimulates the metabolism. However, if your digestion is very weak, it is advisable to follow a food combining programme, at least in the early stages.

As the spleen has an important role to play concerning blood, it is best to ensure that there is a rich supply of good quality 'blood-building' foods in the diet:

- Lycii berries are a Chinese food cure for building blood and supporting the spleen.
- The quality of blood can be improved with foods rich in chlorophyll (the green substance found in leafy green vegetables)
- Beetroot is another excellent food for building blood.
- Other foods which strengthen the blood are apricots, kidney and aduki beans, blue green algae and spirulina, red algae (found in silica formulas), nettles, parsley, watercress, eggs, figs and fish such as sardines.
- Flesh foods are well-known blood builders. TCM has it that if a particular organ is weak, you should eat that organ: liver if your liver needs nourishing, kidneys to boost kidney energy, and so forth. If you decide to follow this principle remember that it is essential with offal, and preferable with other meats too, to buy organic.

Foods *not recommended* because they weaken the blood include:

- Fatty, refined, artificial foods and sweets. Other foods best avoided or eaten in moderation are raw fruit/vegetables, dairy products and sugar, as they create dampness in the spleen.
- Foods not particularly supportive to the spleen are roasted nuts, wheat, yeast, beer and coffee.
- Avoid excessive consumption of cold liquids and concentrated fruit juices, especially tomato or citrus, as they can weaken the spleen.

Helpful herbs and spices

- Ginger is one of the key herbs to strengthen the spleen. Use in hot teas or in cooking.
- Ginseng is recommended as a tonic for the spleen.

- Parsley and celery tea are both excellent drinks to help to dry a damp spleen as they discourage water retention.

Exercise

See pages 28–29.

Touch Therapies

Reflexology

The reflex points for the spleen/pancreas are situated primarily on the left foot. (*See page 30 for massage techniques.*)

Reflexology points for the spleen and pancreas (shaded)

Acupressure

The ancient Chinese grouped the spleen and pancreas together because they are nourished by the same meridian. The spleen-pancreas meridian is in charge of moving and transforming food, then directing and distributing the resultant energy.

There are 21 spleen meridian points, starting on the outside tip of the big toe nail and running along the medial aspect of the foot, up the inside of the leg, to enter the abdomen. The meridian then enters the spleen and stomach, crosses the diaphragm and ends at the centre of the tongue.

SPLEEN 6

This is the most important of all spleen points and is used in spleen deficiency patterns that lead to poor appetite, loose stools and tiredness. However, it can stimulate labour and so *must not be used on pregnant women.*

This point is, more often than not, very tender to the touch and therefore easy to locate. Find the inside of your ankle bone and place three fingers on it; you will find the point above the third finger, just off the edge of the bone. Gently massage the point, or hold it for approximately one minute. Oils will enhance the effect of this treatment.

As it is such a significant point, the benefits are listed below:

- A major point to dry dampness and can help clear related symptoms such as vaginal discharge and itching, mucus in the stool and cloudy urine.
- Has a strong influence on blood and can nourish the blood.
- Excellent for stopping pain, especially abdominal or gynaecological symptoms as it regulates the uterus and menstruation.
- Heavy, painful periods with clotted blood, or scanty periods will be helped by massaging Spleen 6.
- As Spleen 6 is the crossing point of the spleen, liver and kidney, it can be used to promote smooth flow of liver energy and support kidney function.
- Also has a strong calming action on the mind and can help where there is indecision, over-thinking or a 'butterfly' mind.

The spleen meridian

73   *The Spleen*

This point is located below the knee on the inside of the leg, just below the top of the tibia bone. It is often tender when touched. It is helpful where there is water retention in the legs and abdomen as it eliminates excess dampness in the body; also indicated for diarrhoea or loose stools, vaginal discharge and urinary problems.

Spleen 6 (below) and 9 (above) acupressure points

Skin Brushing

Skin brushing is an excellent way to help detoxify the body, as the gentle friction on the skin stimulates the lymphatic system. It is one of the best lymphatic cleansers known, and therefore is supportive to the spleen. When practised daily for a few months it can also improve body tone. This treatment should be carried out on dry skin for about 3 minutes prior to having a shower or bath.

1. Brush the soles as well as the upper sides of the feet using a long-handled natural bristle brush. With long, sweeping strokes, brush up the legs, covering all of the skin's surface area, concentrating on the thighs and buttocks.
2. Put one arm up in the air, allowing gravity to help drain the lymph to the armpit, and sweep down the arm with gentle strokes, drawing the brush towards the armpit.
3. Brush the torso by brushing towards the heart, and when doing the lower abdomen, brush up the right-hand side, just on the inside of the hip bone, across the transverse colon beneath the ribs and down the left-hand side, then gently across the pelvic area to complete the circle. This follows the natural direction of the colon. Repeat.
4. When working near the breast area, brush over the top of the breast, always aiming for the armpit – and remember, be gentle over sensitive areas!

Your skin will become more resilient and you will be able to take more vigorous brushing after a few weeks. Visualize while you do this that your body is being cleansed and purified, with all the toxins being dredged into the lymphatic system to be released in the colon. Stools may contain large amounts of mucus after beginning skin brushing, which is a good sign that the body is beginning to clear away old matter. Skin brushing is subject to 'homeostatic resistance', in other words the body quite simply gets used to it. To override this, it is best to follow a regular daily programme of skin brushing one to two times a day for three months, then reduce this to twice a week – preferably keeping to a regular routine.

Essential Oils

Bitter orange: has an affinity with the spleen and stomach and can help to regulate the *qi* where there is stagnation or symptoms such as abdominal discharge and prolapse. *Strength factor: Medium*

Black pepper: increases production of new red blood cells. Invaluable for anaemia or after heavy blood loss. *Strength factor: Strong*

Benzoin: for lethargy, cold limbs and abdominal bloating. Helps to centre, calm, nourish and comfort those who over-worry. *Strength factor: Weak*

Caraway: helpful for bloating and can alleviate dampness by enhancing the spleen's function of 'transformation'. *Strength factor: Strong*

Fennel: increases the spleen *qi* and stimulates the lymphatic system. Mild diuretic properties, helping to clear congestion and excess weight. Can help the individual who is prone to over-analysing and has a mind that never goes to sleep! *Strength factor: Strong*

Frankincense: good for anyone affected by negative energy or people. Stills the mind, creating peace and calm from within. Has a very strong action on the nervous system and can help to re-build energy levels when they are in danger of weakening the immune system. *Strength factor: Strong*

Ginger: has a real warming and drying effect on the spleen. Both stimulates and tones the digestive system; excellent for abdominal distension, poor appetite, travel sickness (morning sickness too) and nausea. On an emotional level it is good for the Earth personality who can be overwhelmed by self-doubt and over-dependent on others. *Strength factor: Medium*

Lemon: can help to reduce lymphatic congestion, cellulite and obesity. Clears mental sluggishness and strengthens the intellect and mental faculties. Anti-viral properties allow it to support the immune system. A pancreatic stimulant. Can both move the blood and give support to the spleen's function of holding blood and tone in the blood vessels: ideal for haemorrhoids, varicose veins, nose bleeds and even broken capillaries. *Strength factor: Medium*

Marjoram (sweet): both relaxes and gives strength in times of weakness and exhaustion. Can pacify emotional cravings and subdue obsessive thoughts and desires. *Strength factor: Strong*

Myrrh: for those who are lethargic, cold and are congested both mentally and physically. For indolent wounds that don't heal and for vaginal discharges such as thrush. Excellent anti-fungal, anti-bacterial and anti-inflammatory actions. Centres energies, instilling peace and tranquillity to a worried mind. *Strength factor: Medium*

Lavender, Bergamot, Tea tree: stimulate production of white blood cells. *Strength factors: Weak (Lavender), Medium (Bergamot), Strong (Tea Tree)*

Eucalyptus, Rosemary: also act against a wide variety of bacteria and viruses; increase immune response. *Strength factor: Strong*

Emotions

The emotions corresponding to the Earth element are sympathy and worry. The phrase 'I need' will be heard often when this element is out of balance. Emotional manifestations of spleen disorders can be seen in the release of negative, disappointed or selfish feelings together with needy and over-dependent behaviour patterns. Individuals who 'vent their spleen' are often trapped in negative recurring thoughts and feelings for both themselves and others. When there is disharmony with the spleen, there can be feelings of loneliness or antagonism towards the rest of the world.

Worrying is an imbalance in the Earth element and, over time, can develop into obsessional behaviour, mental confusion, dependency and excessive sympathy or pensiveness. This can manifest as the over-protective parent who is constantly worried over his or her children: a 'mother hen' character.

The spleen is said to be the 'residence of thought' or *Yi* and the health of this organ influences our capacity for thinking, studying, concentrating, focusing and memorizing. If the spleen energy is low, this strains the thinking process leading to poor concentration, excessive mental activity, worry and the inability to make decisions.

Flower Remedies

Heather: for individuals who are obsessed with their own troubles, affairs and health issues. Helps them learn to see what lies beyond their personal worries and encourages them to develop greater empathy with others.

Red Chestnut: for those who are over-protective towards their loved ones. Helps them to develop the ability to offer guidance and positive support while still remaining partially detached, so allowing them to experience life without projected worries.

White Chestnut: for those unwanted thoughts that chase around the mind, leaving you exhausted both physically and mentally and unable to focus on important matters. Sleep patterns are always disturbed, with it being particularly difficult to get to sleep due to the incessant chatter of the mind. Instils tranquillity and peace into the very core of your being.

Affirmations

These affirmations can be sung if you prefer, as singing strengthens the spleen!

- My spleen is strong and enables the nourishment of life to reach every part of my body.
- My spleen glows like the warm yellow sunshine, bathing my body in a rejuvenating and healing light.
- My thoughts are calm, my mind is focused and I am at peace.
- My spleen transforms nourishment into golden *qi*, thus increasing my vitality.
- I am at one with Mother Nature and feel safe and secure.

See also the Stomach chapter, page 59, for affirmations that may be used in conjunction with these.

Meditation for the Earth Element
See Stomach chapter, page 49.

The Fire Element

Partner Organs: The organs for the Fire element are the heart and small intestine. The Fire element creates warmth, colour and passion in our lives; when we lack fire, we lack emotional warmth.

Climate: Heat. Excess heat is injurious to the heart. Someone who adores heat or who on the other hand feels extremely uncomfortable in hot weather, may have a Fire imbalance. Hot and painful joints may indicate that fire has got lodged in an area of the body; fevers and thirst, heartburn and hot flushes indicate this as well. Our body heat is on the surface during the Summer, to try to keep us cool and refreshed. Becoming over-heated and having excess fire is one of the main causes of symptoms of imbalance that can arise at this time of year. To compensate, our diet should consist of cooler, lighter foods during hot weather.

Season: Summer, a time when plants have reached their maximum capacity for growth with the hot temperatures and abundant sunshine. We too have more physical energy and often feel the desire to play more sport, do the gardening and go for long walks. It is a time of optimum growth and warmth, like the sun reaching its highest point in the sky. Summer is also an essential time for building and protecting our energy reserves for the remainder of the year. If your energy reserves are low and you feel fatigued, this can mean that the kidney energy is low and that you did not rest enough and recuperate during the Winter. If this is the case, then it is essential that you look after yourself as much as possible in the Summer months, or your energy could be even lower in Winter, leaving you more susceptible to colds and other viral infections.

Colour: Red. When there is a heart imbalance, the skin is highly coloured and have a red tone. A passion for the colour red or, conversely, a total aversion to this colour can point to an imbalance in this element.

Time of Day: 11 a.m.–1 p.m. (heart) and 1–3 p.m. (small intestine).

Body Tissue: The heart controls the blood vessels and blood, regulating and maintaining them. The spleen and liver are also involved with the blood, but the heart provides its rhythm and regulation. (The spleen holds the blood, preventing leakages and haemorrhages, and the liver is responsible for the release and storage of blood.)

Voice Sound: Laughter is the sound for this element: a continuous giggle may be present in the voice, or alternatively there could be a complete absence of laughter and humour. Speech is also ruled by the heart, so incoherence, babbling, stammering and speech impediments, as well as excessive talking, all show that this organ is out of balance.

Sense Organ: The tongue. According to ancient texts, the tongue is the mirror of the heart. A TCM practitioner will pay particular attention to the colour of the tongue and to the state of its tip, as this section of the tongue pertains to the heart. Perspiration is the fluid secretion of Fire; the heart is therefore responsible for our sweat. Note how sweating increases during physical exercise when the heart is beating faster to circulate extra blood and oxygen to the muscles. The ancient Chinese believed that sweat could unclog the body, allowing the body/mind to be cleansed throughout.

Reflector: By looking at the complexion and observing the texture and quality of the skin, the Chinese could read a lot into the state of the Fire element. When the complexion is rosy, the heart is strong; when the face lacks lustre and colour, there may be an imbalance.

Symptoms of Imbalance: Common symptoms that can manifest due to an imbalance include issues around love and self-love, nervous exhaustion or excitability, insomnia, redness and disorders involving the heart.

The Heart

 The heart is a muscle roughly the size of your fist. It is located behind the lungs and is protected by the rib cage.

Western Function

The main function of the heart is to pump oxygen-rich blood around the body through the arteries. Deoxygenated blood is sent back through the veins into the heart, where it is sent to the lungs, the carbon dioxide is expelled and replaced with more oxygen. And so the cycle continues. Half the time is spent in activity (systole or contraction of the heart) and half in relaxation (diastole or resting phase). The vitality and health of the heart and circulatory system are fundamental to life and to the integration of all parts of the body. Any weakness present will, quite naturally, have a profound effect on other organs and tissues in the body. Part of the reason for this is because the circulatory system connects to all other body systems and thus has an impact on them all.

Traditional Chinese Interpretation

Element:	Fire
Partner organ:	Small intestine
Climate:	Heat
Season:	Summer
Colour:	Red
Time of day:	11 a.m.–1 p.m.
Body tissue:	Blood vessels
Voice sound:	Laughter
Sense organ:	Tongue
Reflector:	Complexion
Taste:	Bitter
Emotion:	Joy

SYMPTOMS OF IMBALANCE

Emotional
Anxiety, emotional unease • Forgetfulness • Excessive dreaming • Continuous laughter • Having no joy or humour • Lack of self love • Poor self-esteem • Cruelty, hatred • Over-enthusiasm/agitation • Frigidity • Restlessness

Physical
Hardening of arteries, thrombosis • Heart attacks • Poor circulation • Low blood pressure • High blood pressure • Hot and painful joints • Red face or ashen in colour • Angina • Hot flushes • Weak, irregular pulse • Insomnia • Aversion to heat

---

In Chinese medicine the heart is part of the Fire element and is named Emperor of the Body. According to some sources, the heart determines the state and strength of our constitution. Our constitution is primarily related to the kidney energy, but if the heart is strong and the blood in ample supply and able to circulate freely, then the person will be full of vigour and his or her constitution strong. The lungs play an important supporting role by taking in oxygen and getting rid of carbon dioxide.

According to Chinese medicine, the heart is often seen as the organ most connected with heaven and is described in its spiritual function of 'Housing the Shen'. The concept of the *Shen* is a complex one, there being many interpretations. It is probably best translated as 'spirit', although some authorities interpret the heart as the 'residence of the Mind'. A healthy, vibrant person in good spirits would be described as having a good *Shen* or spirit. The *Shen* is often reflected in shining and twinkling eyes.

Next, taking the *Shen* to translate as 'the mind', mental activity is said to reside in the heart, meaning that the heart will affect our mental and emotional health, in particular our memory, thinking and sleep patterns. If the heart is strong, the mind will be both happy and peaceful, memory and thinking will be sharp, sleep sound and we will be balanced on an emotional level. Insomnia, poor memory (in particular long-term memory of past events), forgetfulness, excessive dreaming and incoherent speech problems can arise if the heart energy is weak.

SELF-HELP FOR KEEPING YOUR HEART HEALTHY

Chinese Nutrition

Foods for the Fire Element

Grain: corn	Fruit: plum
Meat: mutton	Vegetable: coarse greens

The taste corresponding to this element is bitter. The bitter flavour is thought to enter the heart, helping to cool it if it has become overheated as well as cleansing the heart and circulatory system of deposits that have been built up over the years. However, if someone is very weak or deficient, the bitter flavour should be consumed in moderation.

Foods that enhance the Fire function often have colours and qualities that strengthen and stimulate the heart and absorb a lot of sunlight. Such foods include: corn, chives, sunflower seeds, apricots, peaches, plums, red lentils, strawberries and raspberries.

NB It is best to eat foods such as strawberries and other Summer berries only when they are in season.

Dietary Tips

1. Bitter endive, chicory and dandelion are thought to stimulate the heart and small intestine function.
2. Asparagus is a supreme Fire food with a bitter taste and has particularly powerful cleansing properties.
3. Whole grains such as rice and wheat possess bitter qualities in the bran and germ, so it is important to eat them in their natural form, such as brown rice and whole grains.
4. Longan fruit has the appearance of a reddish raisin. It increases the production of blood and comes highly recommended as a cure for insomnia. It has a sweet flavour and so can be used in sweet congees, desserts and soups.

A deficiency of blood in the body can cause many imbalances, as it nourishes our brain, vital organs, muscles and every part of us.

- The quality of blood can be improved through our diet with foods rich in chlorophyll (the green substance found in leafy green vegetables), especially when combined with grains such as millet.
- Beetroot is another excellent food for blood with its rich red colour and high iron content.
- Other foods which strengthen the blood are apricots, kidney and aduki beans, blue-green algae and spirulina, nettles, parsley, watercress, eggs, figs and fish such as sardines.
- Flesh foods are well-documented blood builders and the ancient Chinese believed that if a particular organ was weak, eating the relevant organ from an animal (such as liver if the liver needs building) would help. However, if you decide to follow this principle, it is essential with offal, and preferable with other meats, to buy organic.

To compensate for hot temperatures in Summer, our diet should be of a cooler, lighter nature. Choosing foods which are easy to digest is important. This is the best time of year to eat salads and fresh fruits which are locally grown and in season. However, those individuals who feel cold on a hot day must try and resist the inclination to eat raw foods, salads and ice cream. If you have a weak immune system, eating these cold, damp foods can encourage the formation of mucus in the Autumn.

As an element, Fire is injured by too much spicy food, animal fat and cholesterol in the blood. Red meat, eggs, dairy food and sugar are all known to raise blood cholesterol levels and prevent an adequate supply of oxygen in the blood reaching the heart. The consumption of these should be greatly reduced or avoided when cholesterol levels are high.

The nightshade family (pepper, aubergines, tobacco, tomatoes and potatoes) are thought to weaken the heart, especially if eaten in a cold, damp climate, like we have here in the UK! They are thought to produce high levels of toxic calcium, which lead to circulation problems such as cold hands and feet. If excess alcohol is consumed with these foods, gout, rheumatism and arthritis can develop. The nightshade group also contains the toxin solanine which may cause symptoms of pain, discomfort and arthritis in susceptible individuals.

Calming foods

As the *Shen* or spirit is ruled by the heart, it is important to recognize both the foods which settle and support the *Shen*, and those which can it. Sugar, alcohol, tea, coffee, refined foods, large evening meals and food consumed late at night, as well as an excessive amount of ingredients in a meal can all unsettle the *Shen*. Conversely, lemons have a calming action on the mind, as do whole grains such as rice, oats and wheat. The latter are known for their powerful effect on calming the mind; this is attributed to the fact that these carbohydrate foods raise serotonin levels, an important neurotransmitter in the brain which is known to promote sound sleep and tranquillity. Any food rich in vital minerals, especially calcium, magnesium and silicon, induce a calming action on the spirit.

Foods rich in *calcium* include:

- chlorophyll greens such as watercress, sorrel, rocket, kale, broccoli, parsley, mustard and dandelion greens
- almonds, sesame seeds (and tahini), brazil nuts, sunflower seeds, pumpkin seeds,
- dried figs, pulses, beans, lentils
- white fish, canned salmon and sardines (including the bones)
- olives and oatstraw tea
- soup made with organic meat or fish bones, with green vegetables and a tablespoon of vinegar added – the addition of vinegar helps to draw the calcium out of the bones. Eggshells can be added and removed with the bones before serving!
- milk is technically high in calcium, but the calcium found in dairy foods comes in an unbalanced relationship with the minerals phosphorous and magnesium, which results in inefficient assimilation and absorption. The nightshade group of vegetables, mentioned earlier, together with citrus fruits can negatively affect calcium balance in the body. Wine, salt and vinegar should be consumed in moderation as these too can bring about a loss of calcium in the body. Fizzy drinks, including carbonated water, lead to excess levels of phosphorus, so disrupting the natural balance of calcium, magnesium and phosphorus, which can result in bone loss.

Foods rich in *magnesium* include:

- green vegetables rich green chlorophyll (*see calcium list, above, for examples*)
- kelp
- millet, brown rice
- dried apricots and peaches, bananas, dates, avocado, raisins
- lentils, peas and beans, cashews and black walnuts.

Foods rich in *silicon* include:

- lettuce, celery, asparagus, dandelion greens, horseradish, spinach, leeks, artichokes, celery, alfalfa, mustard greens
- strawberries, apples, carrots, watermelon and cucumber
- rice, sunflower seeds, sea vegetables.

Fish oils are extremely beneficial to the heart and the whole body as they provide omega 3 fatty acids. You should have at least two portions a week of oily fish such as salmon and mackerel. Another source of omega 3 fatty acids is linseed oil, which is ideal for vegetarians. Virgin cold-pressed vegetable and seed oils provide valuable omega 6 fatty acids which, like the omega 3 fatty acids, are vital for brain function, hormones and general health. Sudden weight loss regimes and diets must be discouraged as they are particularly harmful to the heart and can put it under great strain. It is common sense to lower the amounts of saturated fats in the diet by choosing lean meats and lower fat products and also to cut down on the amount of hidden fats in the diet – as found in cakes, pastries and biscuits.

Moderation is always the key, so ensure your diet is varied and enjoyable!

Helpful herbs and spices
- Chamomile and mint herb teas can help to clear excess heat and have a soothing and relaxing effect on the body.
- Dill and basil have a calming effect on the body; the latter is also thought to be unrivalled in its ability to enhance memory and promote clear concentration.
- Garlic is well-known for its positive effects on the heart and circulatory system.
- A small amount of cayenne pepper is excellent for the heart and circulation; also enhances the thorough digestion of foods.
- Mung bean tea is another simple yet highly effective way of lowering blood pressure. Pour hot water over 2 tablespoons of washed mung beans and drink first thing in the morning. Keep the mung beans and pour another 240 ml of hot water over at lunch time and drink. Save the beans yet again, pour another 240 ml of hot water over the beans and drink in the evening. Mung beans can also be cooked and added to soups or salads.
- Cassia seed can be purchased from a Chinese pharmacy. It has a similar taste to coffee and has the unique ability to bring blood pressure down. It also strengthens eyesight and clears vision. Pan roast and grind into a powder and mix a teaspoon with 240 ml of hot water.

- Lotus seeds have the ability to relax the mind and calm the spirit. They can be added to soups, stews and congees.

In hot countries, hot spices such as black pepper, red and green chillies and ginger are consumed for a good reason. These are dispersing spices, which open the pores and take heat out of the body, by encouraging sweating. They are ultimately cooling foods in the body, although their taste may at first tell you quite differently!

Exercise

Exercise that is of a moderate intensity and adequate enough to get the heart rate up for 30–40 minutes three times a week is recommended to strengthen the heart and cardiovascular system. Deep breathing techniques, visualization, meditation, massage and acupressure are examples of the effective methods available which can help to calm and settle the *Shen*.

The exercise to stretch the heart and small intestine meridians begins by sitting on the floor with your knees open and the soles of the feet together. Keeping your back straight, inhale and gently lean forward. Exhale as you move into the stretch, seeing if you can lower your knees a little nearer to the floor and bring your head towards your feet. The objective is to try and bring your head, elbows and knees as close as possible to the floor. Remember that it may take many weeks or months to achieve this. Always work at your own pace and ensure that you have warmed the muscles in your body for 10 minutes prior to stretching. If possible, join a local yoga class where you can be guided and personally instructed.

The heart/small intestine stretch

Touch Therapies

Massage

Massaging the sternum close to the heart can help to release tension and tightness around the chest area and ease difficult breathing. Starting at the top of the sternum, work down in small spirals until you reach the tip of the sternum, spending more time on congested, sore areas. For particularly sore points or if you feel emotional pain while doing this exercise, make the sound 'HAWWWWWW', which strengthens the heart, and visualize the colour pink or green, whichever you feel intuitively is more suitable. You can also get someone to hold the tip of your sternum and acupressure point Heart 7 for a few minutes. 9–11 a.m. is a particularly potent time to work on issues pertaining to the heart.

Using your eyes excessively, as when working at a desk for long hours, can weaken the heart and small intestine meridians, as can emotional stress, which can go on to create more emotional imbalances. One of the best points to help return equilibrium is CV17 (The Sea of Tranquillity). This is at the centre of your sternum (breastbone) and often feels tender. As with the stretch for the Fire element, visualizing the colour pink can help to ease tension and anxiety stored in this area, as can making the heart sound 'HAWWWWWW' while gently massaging this point.

Reflexology

The reflex point for the heart is on the ball of the left foot. Never over-stimulate this reflex, instead gently massage the whole area indicated in the diagram. (*See page 30 for massage techniques.*)

Reflexology point for the heart (shaded)

Acupressure

The heart meridian has nine points. It originates at the heart although the first official point (Heart 1) is located under both arms. It runs down the inner arm andt finishes on the inside of the nail bed of the little finger nail (Heart 9). It controls the thyroid and influences many menopausal symptoms, such as hot flushes.

The heart meridian

HEART 7

This is the most important point on the heart channel and one of the major acupressure points on the body. Its main action is to calm the mind; it is also used to stimulate poor memory, ease palpitations and anxiety and alleviate insomnia. It is a truly excellent point to calm an over-active, worried mind and to take the heat out of stressful situations.

Heart 7 is located on the inside of the wrist, on the crease. Cupping your wrist, with one hand gently rub the point using your thumb, or alternatively, gently hold the point for approximately one minute. Breathe deeply while you do this, feeling peace and tranquillity flowing into your body and soul.

Heart 7 (on the wrist) and Heart 9 (on the little finger) acupressure points

HEART 9

This point can be massaged to calm excess heart heat which has symptoms such as dry mouth, night sweats, insomnia and mental restlessness. Even just massaging the general location of the point on the fingertip by the nail bed is beneficial, as is holding the point between your thumb and finger of your other hand.

It is thought that Heart 7 is more effective on men than women, and that women respond better to a point on the heart protector or pericardium channel, Pericardium 7. Pericardium 6 is another major acupuncture point and is one of the best body points to enhance our ability to relate to the outside world, ourselves and our partners. This 'spirit point', as it is known, regulates the energy and protects the heart and can help support us in our personal relationships where the heart may have got 'emotionally' injured as a result of difficulties relating to our loved ones.

Pericardium 6 (on the wrist) and 7 (under the thumb) acupressure points

PERICARDIUM 6

This is located in the middle of the inside of the forearm, approximately two and a half finger-widths away from the wrist crease. Gently hold the point for approximately one minute and feel your anxiety and stress levels diminish.

PERICARDIUM 7

This point is located on the inside of the wrist, on the mid-point of the crease. Cupping your wrist, with one hand gently rub the point using your thumb, or alternatively, gently hold the point for approximately one minute and feel your anxieties leaving your body. This point is very powerful aid to comforting and supporting emotions when there are relationship problems. Working on Pericardium 6 and 7 together can enhance the beneficial results.

Essential Oils

Jasmine: a beautiful, sensual oil which is very relaxing and emotionally warming. Eases depression and apathy. Helps with relationship problems where sexual difficulties such as frigidity and impotence are involved. Restores confidence and is a good choice for someone with low self-esteem. *Strength factor: Strong*

Lavender: has an affinity with the Fire element, partly due to its ability to clear heat. On an emotional level calms and soothes the *Shen* in times of stress and exhaustion, so helping with symptoms such as panic attacks, hysteria and insomnia. Invokes peacefulness of spirit and tranquillity of the mind. Can lower blood pressure and ease palpitations. *Strength factor: Weak*

Neroli: calms anxiety, nervousness, hysteria and shock; uplifts the *Shen*. Restores feelings of joy to those who have suffered deep emotional pain. Well indicated for palpitations and high blood pressure; has a cleansing and purifying action on the blood. *Strength factor: Strong*

Palmarosa: useful for emotional burnout and nervous tension. Calms palpitations, insomnia and restlessness. *Strength factor: Medium*

Rose: one of the most powerful aromatherapy oils for the issues around love; enhances love of the self when we have over-extended ourselves in life. *Strength factor: Strong*

Rosemary: promotes circulation, strengthens the heartbeat and raises low blood pressure. Refreshing and stimulating, Rosemary is thought to help with speech impediments (which

are connected to the heart and to a Fire imbalance). Can also increase the supply of blood to the brain, and thus has a reputation as an invigorating brain tonic.
Strength factor: Strong

Ylang ylang: a renowned sexual tonic and aphrodisiac often chosen to help with sexual problems such as impotence and frigidity. Helps with palpitations, rapid heart beat, high blood pressure, depression, anxiety, restlessness and lack of joy.
Strength factor: Strong

Emotions

Dis-ease is often viewed as a sign that we are becoming more out of harmony with nature. As the heart spends equal time in activity and relaxation, it is important to assess your lifestyle patterns and see if you spend half of your time relaxing and half working. If you don't, it is important to re-evaluate your situation.

Joy is the emotion associated with the heart and the Fire element. Joy in the positive embodies enthusiasm, fun, happiness and laughter. The Chinese in their wisdom, however, realized that the emotion of joy, either in excess or deficiency, could be just as detrimental to our health as excessive anger. Permanent joy is an impossible thirst and, if sought after through work or play, can put too much stress on the system. In the homoeopathic Materia Medica, excess joy is termed 'mania'. It can agitate the *Shen* or spirit, so triggering insomnia, anxiety, palpitations and other heart problems. Some say that too much joy means a suppression of the other emotions, which all play a part in our make-up – anger, grief, fear and reflection, and that excess joy at inappropriate moments demonstrates a disharmony of the heart.

Heart troubles can reflect our 'emotional heart', be it lack of self-love, lack of love as a child, difficulties with parents, problems with a loved one in a relationship, etc. Bringing more love into our lives and loving ourselves a little more can go a long way towards helping us to cope with stress.

Flower Remedies

Agrimony: for those who on the surface may appear cheerful but underneath are hiding anxiety and mental torture. Can transform inner pain and suffering by bringing a note of lightness, joy and the ability to laugh at our problems.

White Chestnut: for those suffering from insomnia due to unwanted thoughts racing around their head at night. Helps to quiet and calm mental processes, thus allowing the mind to function more efficiently and clearly. Instils an air of tranquillity; can be used to bring about a state of peace and harmony, thus settling the *Shen*.

You may also find some appropriate remedies for supporting the Fire element in the chapter on the small intestine (page 110).

Affirmations

- My heart joyfully pumps blood to every living cell in my body.
- My heart beats happily with the rhythm of life.
- I fill my heart with peace and joy which I can now share with others.
- I am a loving person who attracts loving relationships.
- I love myself.
- Joy and love fill my body and soul.

See also the Small Intestine chapter, page 99, for affirmations that may be used in conjunction with these.

Meditation for the Fire Element

Before beginning this meditation, familiarize yourself with the diagrams of the relevant meridians (i.e. for the heart and small intestine). Remember that *qi* is pronounced 'chee', and that all meridians are bilateral (running along both sides of the body); for the purposes of this meditation the meridian points on only one side of the body are focused on. If possible, tape this meditation, reading it out clearly and slowly in a soft tone of voice.

Find a peaceful place to relax and unwind. Close your eyes. Focus your attention on your breathing and, as you begin to notice it deepening, gently let any thoughts that come into your mind float by like clouds in the sky. For a few minutes, practise the breathing exercise recommended in the Lung chapter (*page 183*).

Fire Meditation

Imagine yourself lying on a beach on a beautiful Summer's day. The sky is azure blue and the sun radiates warmth and light deep into your body. In the background you can hear the gentle sound of waves as they roll onto the shore. Breathe the warmth and light of the sun and feel it strengthening and nourishing your body. Allow this energy to flow down to your heart and see your heart being supported by a beautiful soft pink colour. Feel the healing that this colour brings to your heart; sense it calming your heart and settling your spirit.

Feel peace and tranquillity flowing through you and easing any stress or tension held in your body. See your heart getting stronger and healthier every day, and the pink energy strengthening your circulation and encouraging your blood to flow freely. Feel your capacity to give unconditional love expand and fill your own heart with love and joy. Visualize the Heart meridian emerging from your heart, flowing to your left armpit and travelling down the inside of your arm until it reaches your little finger. Send energy down this channel and feel it dissolving any congestion in the meridian.

Then channel the energy into your Small Intestine meridian, which runs up the outside of your arm, across your shoulder, up your neck and around your ear to its finishing point in front of your ear. Now, send energy down to your small intestine and allow it to cleanse and purify this area. The warm, pink energy will enhance the small intestine's ability to separate the pure from the impure. This strengthens your ability in life to unleash your true powers of discrimination, so making confused thinking and indecisiveness things of the past.

Visualize the area in your lower abdomen becoming stronger and believe that your small intestine has the ability to assimilate and absorb necessary nutrients. Feel waves of pink energy washing over your whole body, filling your mind, body and spirit with a deep sense of joy and fulfilment. Sense your energy becoming stronger and begin to move your fingers and toes, feeling yourself becoming more alive and awake ... and, in your own time, open your eyes and stretch your body out.

NB You can visualize the colour red rather than pink, but the effects will be stronger. If you have any symptoms of inflammation or heat in the body, choose pink; if you have very poor circulation and are very cold, then try using the colour red instead.

The Small Intestine

 The small intestine is a long, thin tube about 7 metres long; it lies at the base of the stomach and coils through the central and lower area of the abdomen to join with the colon.

Western Function

The small intestine participates in all aspects of digestion, including the absorption and transportation of food. It produces enzymes which combine with those sent by the pancreas and gallbladder to help break food down into smaller components. Proteins are thus converted into amino acids, carbohydrates are broken down into simple sugars, and fats into smaller units, allowing efficient absorption to take place.

The inner surface of the small intestine is covered with tiny finger-like projections called *villi* which increase the area available for absorption. They act like a filter, helping to prevent toxins from being reabsorbed back into the body. Smaller particles of food go through this lining to the liver via the portal vein system, where substances are further processed before reaching the rest of the body. If the small intestine becomes too full of toxins, it can slow the speed and efficiency of the digestive system and impair absorption, as a congested intestine cannot perform all its physiological functions.

One such absorption disorder is coeliac's disease which is caused by an allergy to gluten, the sticky protein found in many grains including wheat. The intestinal lining and villi become damaged and defective, causing serious malabsorption problems and resulting in losses of vitamins and minerals, with diarrhoea compounding the problem. Key symptoms include nausea, smelly stools, abdominal distension, body pain, skin rashes and weight loss.

The quality of our blood – that is, the extent to which it receives adequate nutrition – depends on our diet and the functioning of the small intestine. As the small intestine absorbs iron from our food, which helps to transport oxygen to the cells around the body, it follows that if iron levels are low there will be a corresponding drop in the oxygen-carrying capacity of the blood.

Traditional Chinese Interpretation

Element:	Fire
Partner organ:	Heart
Climate:	Heat
Season:	Summer
Colour:	Red
Time of day:	1–3 p.m.
Body tissue:	Blood vessels
Voice sound:	Laughter
Sense organ:	Tongue
Reflector:	Complexion
Taste:	Bitter
Emotion:	Joy

SYMPTOMS OF IMBALANCE

Emotional
Sadness • Mental confusion • Lack of joy • Critical and cynical •
Naive and gullible • Over-thinking • Ambitious but fails to
appreciate success • Unable to separate pure from impure

Physical
Poor muscle tone in abdomen • Pain in lower abdomen, throat or
shoulder • Stiff neck and a double chin • Abscesses in the mouth
and upper lip • Tennis elbow, frozen shoulder • Difficulty turning
head 180 degrees • Hearing difficulties • Urinary problems •
Haemorrhoids and varicose veins • Coeliac's disease • Anaemia

In Chinese medicine, the two main functions of the small intestine
are to 'separate fluids' and to control 'receiving and transforming'.
The small intestine receives fluids and food from the stomach
after digestion, then 'transforms' these by separating the 'pure'
from the 'impure': the clean and usable parts of the food from
parts no longer needed. The 'impure' parts are sent to the bladder
to be released as urine, while the 'clean' parts are sent to the large
intestine, not for excretion, but so that vital fluids are reabsorbed
into the system. The small intestine has, therefore, a direct and
functional relationship with the bladder (which is why bladder
problems are included in the 'Symptoms of Imbalance' above).

The small intestine transforms food in coordination with the
spleen and the kidneys, although it is important to stress that
the small intestine's role is subordinate.

When energy in the small intestine is depleted, you often
encounter absorption difficulties and possible malnutrition.
Lower back problems can develop, especially around the *hara*
area (located between the pubic bone and navel, and known in
Eastern cultures as the source of vitality and health) and there is
likely to be fatigue in the hips and legs. Intestinal disorders can
also lead to headaches and migraines.

Conversely, too much energy in the small intestine can give
rise to stiffness in the neck region in the morning. There is a

coldness in the *hara* due to poor circulation in the lower organs. Cold extremities is another common symptom, as are frequent urination and constipation alternating with diarrhoea.

SELF-HELP FOR KEEPING YOUR SMALL INTESTINE HEALTHY

Chinese Nutrition

Foods for the Fire Element

Grain: corn	Fruit: plum
Meat: mutton	Vegetable: coarse

Dietary Tips

1. The taste corresponding to this element is bitter, so bitter endive, chicory and dandelion stimulate the functioning of the small intestine.
2. Asparagus is a supreme Fire food with particularly powerful cleansing properties, as you can often tell from the strong smell of urea in the urine after eating this vegetable.

The Fire element is injured by too much spicy food, animal fats and cholesterol in the blood. Too much fat and cholesterol can coat the tiny villi of the small intestine, preventing them from being able to filter nutrients properly. The consequences of this are that the cells in the surrounding area will become under-nourished. Excessive consumption of hot and spicy foods can ultimately create heat in the small intestine; conversely, too much raw food can contribute towards coldness in the small intestine.

Diet is of extreme importance to the small intestine, which transforms food using a variety of secretions, including enzymes, to break down various components of food into smaller parts to allow for proper absorption. These secretions are mainly produced in the intestine and only remain present when the diet is harmonious and consists of natural foods. If the diet is high in artificial and commercially prepared products then the valuable intestinal flora population can decline. Acidophilus, a beneficial bacteria found in natural 'live' yoghurt, can be added to the diet to help maintain levels of valuable intestinal flora.

If the small intestine is very congested, you should eat boiled white rice for two to three days, ensuring that you chew each mouthful between 50 and 100 times. As already mentioned, 'live' yoghurt and acidophilus powder are helpful too and can heal and soothe the small intestine. Once you have started the detoxification process you will be able to do some gentle massage over the small intestine area.

Refer to the heart chapter (*page 81*) for more information on foods that support the Fire element.

Exercise

The specific exercise to stretch the heart and small intestine meridians is described on page 89.

Touch Therapies

Massage

The area of a healthy small intestine can be covered with one spread hand and should feel soft and even to the touch. If you press down lightly, it should move gently. If it is full of toxins, there will be a real lack of tone together with an enlargement of the abdomen. Some parts will be slack, others tight, and there will be an uneven quality about the area as it is filled with gas and liquid. This can press downwards and disturb the blood flow in the lower abdomen, resulting in menstrual disorders, varicose veins and haemorrhoids. This excess weight bends the curve of the lower back, pressing on the nerves of the lumbar and sacral plexus, thus inhibiting the messages that the nerves should be getting from the lower abdominal area and organs. This creates muscular tension in the back and legs and can pull at the diaphragm, causing a contraction of the muscles around the ribs. This can create mucus in the lungs and weakens the lymphatic system through lack of movement in the abdomen, thus creating a vicious cycle of toxicity and tension.

Massaging the small intestine helps to eliminate congestion and allows for the smooth flow of energy together with improved digestion and elimination.

If the abdomen feels very hard and painful to the touch, work on it only very gently. You may feel knots in the small intestine: these can build up pressure against the nerves that come out of the spine, and contribute to tight muscles. This results in painful contractions of muscles, nerves, lymph and blood vessels. Do not work on these knots directly, but gently massage the area first to loosen it, then add a little more pressure directly to the knotty area itself.

Using your eyes excessively as when working at a desk for long hours, or emotional stress, can weaken both the heart and small intestine meridians, which can then go on to create more emotional imbalances. One of the best points to help return balance and equilibrium is CV17 (known as the Sea of Tranquillity). This is located at the centre of your sternum or breastbone. It will probably feel tender to the touch, so gently massage the area using the tips of your fingers in a circular motion. Although the colour for the Fire element is red, I would advise visualizing the colour pink to help ease tension and anxiety in this area. As you work on this point, try making the heart sound, 'HAWWWWWW'.

Breathing is of the utmost importance to help improve circulation in this area. Place one hand on your navel and the other hand on your chest. Inhale, gently, filling your body like a balloon with air, distending your abdomen like a pregnant woman. If you are breathing correctly, the hand on your abdomen should rise while the one on your chest should remain quite still. Hold the breath for a few moments and then release it, smoothly and calmly, imagining that any tension and toxins are being released with the exhalation.

Reflexology

The reflex point for the small intestine is found on both feet. Reflexologists tend to 'walk' their thumb across this area diagonally or to work from the outer edge of the foot towards the inside in straight lines. (*See page 30 for massage techniques.*)

Reflexology points for the small intestine (shaded)

The small intestine meridian

Acupressure

The small intestine meridian starts on the outer edge of the little fingernail bed, runs up the outer arm behind the elbow, dips over the back of the shoulder to the cheekbone and ends just in front of the ear.

Small Intestine 3 acupressure point

SMALL INTESTINE 3

Massaging this point is excellent for relieving a stiff neck, occipital headache, aches down the spine and back. It has a deep effect on the muscles and tendons along the course of the governing vessel and bladder channel, as well as the small intestine channel.

It is located on the outer edge of the hand, approximately one finger-width down from the base of the little finger, just beneath the joint. Support your hand at the wrist and, using the thumb of your other hand, massage or hold the point firmly for one minute.

It can clear dampness and also clears the mind, allowing you to make correct and proper choices, as well as giving you the strength to face difficulties in life.

Essential Oils

Bitter orange: anti-spasmodic; aids relaxation and can both decongest and tonify. Ideal for symptoms of abdominal distension and pain. Instils an air of buoyancy and joy when inhaled. *Strength factor: Medium*

Black pepper: increases local circulation and stimulates a sluggish digestive system. Eases pain and spasm. Restores tone to the muscles of the intestines and can aid digestion of heavy food stuffs. *Strength factor: Strong*

Chamomile: possesses anti-inflammatory properties and relieves symptoms of spasm and discomfort in the small intestine, making it an ideal oil for coeliac's disease. *Strength factor: Strong*

Cypress: decongests and detoxifies. Due to its astringent properties it helps to constrict and give tone to the veins. *Strength factor: Medium*

Marjoram: releases tension knots and tangles in the small intestine. Eases muscular spasm in the lower back. Increases blood flow and promotes circulation, helping to decongest the small intestine while at the same time soothing and relaxing the area. *Strength factor: Strong*

Emotions

The heart is the partner organ of the small intestine; it is on the psychological level that you can see the closeness of this partnership. The heart governs the whole of our mental life and the small intestine rules our capacity to be clear about our judgements and decision-making.

In Oriental medicine, the small intestine is in charge of digesting emotions as well as food, and is known as the Abdominal Brain. The small intestine meridian is a receiving and assimilating vessel involved with nourishment at all levels – emotional, mental and spiritual.

Confusion in our mental state is a common symptom which can arise if the small intestine is unable to sort out the 'pure' from the 'impure'. We will have trouble making clear choices and differentiating between good judgement and poor judgement. This can manifest on a physical level in hearing difficulties (an inability to 'sort out' sounds). The gallbladder is also a decision-maker and, if weak, leads to a lack of courage or conviction to carry decisions through. If the small intestine is weak, however, a decision cannot be made in the first place, as we lose the ability to sort through information or to distinguish between the various options and arrive at a sensible decision. There is possibly no more important role in our lives than to see what is of value and use it to our advantage. What is pure and what is impure, and what are our priorities?

When the small intestine is not in balance an individual becomes ambivalent and is unable to commit to a career, relationship or indeed any course of action that could be sustaining and nourishing. This can ultimately lead to self-doubt and frustration as talents are wasted and opportunities lost. Emotions can swing between being overly critical and cynical to, conversely, being naive and gullible. People with a weak small intestine also think too much and control their emotions with their minds; as a result they can experience a deep sense of sadness and lack of joy. If there is excess energy in the small intestine, individuals will be restless, drive themselves hard, overwork, eat fast, find it impossible to relax and will suppress their emotions. They are highly ambitious but often fail to appreciate their accomplishments.

According to ancient Oriental beliefs, negative emotions are expressed in the small intestine by the contraction of particular parts of this organ. Anger contracts the right side of the intestine near the liver; worry affects the upper left side near the spleen; impatience affects the top of the intestine; sadness affects both the lateral sides; fear affects the deeper and lower areas.

Flower Remedies

Cerato: for people who doubt their own judgement and feel they cannot make a valid decision without asking for help from someone else.

Scleranthus: for those who just cannot make up their mind and are easily thrown into a state of confusion. Such people are constantly vacillating – even their moods can alternate from happy to sad. Scleranthus fosters clarity of thought and opens us up to our natural wisdom to light and guide our way.

Vervain: for those who suffer from excessive small intestine energy leading to a pattern of over-work coupled with a driving ambition which does not allow them to relax or appreciate their accomplishments.

Wild Oat: for those who are unable to commit to a career, relationship or any future course of action. Wild Oat is for those with many available opportunities but find themselves unable to decide which path to follow.

Affirmations

- My small intestine joyfully absorbs all the nutrients that I need to keep my body healthy.
- I am able to assimilate nourishment on every level of my being.
- I think clearly, wisely and decisively on all levels.

See also the Heart chapter, page 96, for affirmations that may be used in conjunction with these.

Meditation for the Fire Element
See Heart chapter, page 97.

The Water Element

Partner Organs: The bladder and kidneys are paired together – theirs is perhaps the most obvious of all coupled relationships. In both Western and ancient Eastern physiological understanding, the kidneys and bladder are connected both structurally and functionally. They make up the watergate of the body, as the bladder collects urine excreted by the kidneys and holds it until it leaves the body, thus regulating the flow of water.

Climate: The Water element is connected to the North, so it is not surprising that the climate associated with it is cold. Low temperatures and damp conditions can exacerbate and even cause many symptoms pertaining to this element. The kidney energy, like that of the lungs, can be more vulnerable and open to the cold if we have not taken proper care of ourselves over the Summer. People with a weak Water element generally hate the Winter and really feel the cold. Maintaining your body temperature and wearing appropriate clothing in the Winter months are essential. Make sure you keep your home well heated and be aware that sudden exposure to extreme cold is depleting to the system. Protecting the kidney area is also of vital importance: a scarf worn round your waist will work wonders for your energy over Winter and can protect your kidney 'fire'.

Season: Winter. A person with a Water imbalance could experience an aggravation of symptoms in cold weather or may simply detest the Wintertime. Winter is a time for conserving energy, an important part of restoring balance in this vital element, as is proper nourishment, warmth and rest. It is a time of consolidation, of going inwards and hibernating! Psychologically, it is a time of reflection, to contemplate on the year gone by, to assess whether we have met our goals and what lessons we have learned. As symptoms can become more pronounced in Winter, this season can be difficult for some to cope with as the cold can settle deep into the system. Simple advice is to keep warm, rest as much as possible and eat nourishing, warm foods.

Colour: Dark blue, although traditionally the colour associated with the kidneys is black, or blue/black. There may be a bluish-black tinge to the skin on the face, especially beneath the eyes, which is the area of the face representing the kidneys, together with puffiness if there is an imbalance in the kidneys. Someone who prefers blue and likes to wear it, or conversely has a strong dislike for the colour, may have an imbalance of the Water element.

Time of Day: 3–5 p.m. (bladder); a person with a Water imbalance may find that this corresponds to the time of day when they feel most anxious, tired or irritable. Conversely, if this is your best time of day this too could indicate a slight imbalance, as bladder energy may be in excess. Usually during this time, if there is an urgency to urinate, the body is saying that it wants to let go of the wastes of the day. The time of the kidneys is 5–7 p.m., which may correspond to your lowest energy point in the day with feelings of fatigue and lethargy. If your kidneys are weak, this is a good time of day to rest or meditate.

Body Tissue: The kidneys are in charge of the bones and marrow, which means that all bones including the spine, teeth and skull are kept strong and rigid by the energy sent to them by the Water element. Low kidney energy can result in soft or brittle bones, weak legs and knees and stiffness of the spine, as both bone development and repair depend on the health of the kidneys. The marrow is included as part of the bones, as are the spinal cord and the brain, which is known as the 'sea of marrow'.

Voice Sound: Moaning. When there is an imbalance in the Water element, the affected person cannot help but complain, moan and groan about life's little problems; their feelings are clearly detected in their voice.

Sense Organ: The ear. Hearing problems are often connected to weak kidney energy.

Reflector: The external manifestation of the Water element is the hair, so a glossy, healthy head of hair shows us that the kidney energy is strong. Conversely, if the hair is dry, broken or split, lacks lustre, goes grey too early or starts thinning or falling out, this reflects weak kidney energy.

Symptoms of Imbalance: Key words for the Water element are fluidity and flow. Any imbalance of our body/mind linked to fluid, such as dryness or thirst, excess or lack of perspiration, urination difficulties, feelings of being overwhelmed or tearful, lymphatic congestion, swelling and bloating, lack of sexual secretions, etc. demonstrate that the kidneys are not functioning as they should. The kidneys nourish the brain and influence short-term memory in everyday life. When there is a decline in kidney energy as we grow older, the brain does not receive sufficient nourishment. This can lead to memory loss. Learning difficulties also manifest when kidney energy is low. If marrow production is impaired in any way then it can lead to blood deficiency, blurred vision, hearing difficulties and tinnitus. The lower back area is considered by TCM to be the 'Palace of the kidneys', and so a lack of kidney energy may lead to low back pain and pains in the legs.

The bladder is part of the Water element so the blood and lymphatics also play a significant role as they are all systems that move fluid around the body. Urinary function, perspiration, saliva and tears are all influenced by the Water element.

The Bladder

The bladder is a hollow muscular bag located in the lower abdomen and is connected to the kidneys via a pair of tubes called the ureters.

Western Function

The urinary system, which consists of the bladder, the kidneys and the urethra, is one of the body's main methods of elimination. The bladder is in charge of storing and controlling the release of urine, which is excreted from the kidneys. The bladder is able to expand and contract easily due to its elastic muscle fibres, and can hold about 750 ml of liquid. As fluid collects inside the bladder, it builds up pressure until you feel the desire to go to the lavatory.

Traditional Chinese Interpretation

Element:	Water
Partner organ:	Kidneys
Climate:	Cold
Season:	Winter
Colour:	Blue/black
Time of day:	3–5 p.m.
Body tissue:	Bones and marrow
Voice sound:	Moaning
Sense organ:	Ears
Reflector:	Head hair
Taste:	Salty
Emotion:	Fear

SYMPTOMS OF IMBALANCE

Emotional
Armouring, emotional strain • Complaining • Moaning • Highly sensitive • Fears of inundation • Lack of flow in thought processes and emotions • Crying spells • Deep depression • Fear • Feelings of suspicion

Physical
Poor bladder control and function • Muscular tension running up the back • Tightness in back of the legs and hips • Coolness along the spine and buttocks • Dull, throbbing headache • Poor circulation • Sciatica or lumbago • Cystitis and bladder infections • Pale copious urine or scanty and dark • Lack of perspiration; dryness and thirst • Stiffness in little toe • Brittleness of joints • Spasms or pains in calves • Nosebleeds • Headaches at back or top of head

---

The bladder is considered to be one of the most sensitive organs in the body. It can react not only to physical stimuli but also to our emotions. Fear and shock (emotions which affect the Water element in Chinese medicine) can stimulate the desire to urinate, as can feeling cold, or standing barefoot on cold floors. Bladder infections, as anyone will know who has suffered them, make you aware of the desire to urinate frequently although there is little joy in the amount of urine that is actually passed!

The bladder is an important detoxification and elimination organ; the kidney provides the necessary *qi* to support bladder function. If there is a lack of kidney *qi*, symptoms such as retention of urine or difficulty in urinating can arise. If the bladder is not in balance, any aspect of fluidity within our body/mind may go awry, as Fluidity and Flow are the key words for the Water element. Symptoms such as brittleness of joints, dryness and thirst, frequency or indeed infrequency of urination, excess or deficiency of perspiration, the lack of flow in thought processes and emotions, and feelings or fears of inundation and being overwhelmed by life can arise. Adaptability is a key bladder characteristic on many levels, part of the process of flow within the entire mind/body/spirit. If the bladder is not functioning efficiently, the rest of our system will be greatly stressed. In Chinese medicine, excessive sex is said to deplete the kidney energy, and as the bladder is related to the kidneys, this may explain the occurrence of 'honeymoon cystitis'.

SELF-HELP FOR KEEPING YOUR BLADDER HEALTHY

Chinese Nutrition

Foods for the Water Element

Grain: beans and peas	Fruit: dates
Meat: pork	Vegetable: sea vegetables

Other foods that strengthen the Water element are:

- kidney beans and aduki beans
- barley and buckwheat
- sea vegetables such as kombu, wakame and nori.

See the chapter on the kidneys (page 129) for further information on foods for the Water element.

As the taste for this element is salty, a small amount of salt is often used in Chinese herbal remedies to direct the remedy down to the kidney/bladder area.

If you have the urge to urinate frequently and there is burning, pain and occasionally blood in the urine, then it is likely that you are suffering from a bladder infection. Cystitis and other bladder infections plague women more often today than any health problem except colds, and are usually caused by bacteria in the urethra and bladder.

Tips to help alleviate cystitis
- Avoid sugar and sweet foods.
- Drink lots of water, as this dilutes the concentration of bacteria in the urine.
- Cranberry juice (approximately 480 ml a day) possesses unique compounds that stop the infectious bacteria from clinging to the cells lining the urinary tract and bladder. Do read labels carefully as some contain high levels of sugar which defeats the object. You can buy an excellent powder which consists of freeze-dried cranberries combined with acidophilus which is highly effective and can also be taken as a preventative measure. You can buy frozen cranberries, but where possible use the fresh fruit.
- Avoid caffeine – curtail consumption of chocolate, which contains caffeine and sugar! Tea and cola drinks also contain caffeine.

If you have difficulty urinating, try some of the following additional food cures:
- Onion and garlic are effective against infections or the urinary tract, as is cider vinegar.

- Mash onion and steam it, then apply as a poultice or hot compress to the abdomen below the navel.
- Try broccoli and cabbage soup. Soups or broths made with aduki beans, celery, carrots, potato skins and asparagus clear dampness and heat from the bladder area.
- Eat peas and spinach.
- Kidney beans promote elimination and are excellent diuretics. For swelling due to kidney disorders, make a strong soup with 50 g beans to 1.2 litres of water, cooked down to 240 ml. *Always* ensure that the beans are cooked thoroughly.

Helpful herbs and spices
- Nettle tea is useful for bladder infections.
- The herb *uva ursi* is very good for cystitis and other infections and can be drunk as a tea.
- Crushed watermelon seeds made into a tea make a useful remedy for the bladder.

Exercise

The stretch for the bladder and kidney meridian involves the muscles at the back of the thighs. Sit on the floor and stretch your legs out in front of you. Do not lock your knees but keep them slightly 'soft'. Keeping your lower back straight, gently stretch forwards taking your hands towards your toes. If you cannot reach your toes, reach to your knees or ankles. Relax into this position and breathe gently and deeply; with each breath, imagine energy moving down your body to the back of your thighs, relaxing the muscles and allowing a deeper stretch. Remember that it may take many weeks or months to achieve this. Always work at your own pace and ensure that you have warmed the muscles in your body for 10 minutes prior to stretching. If possible, join a local yoga class where you can be guided and personally instructed. *(See diagram overleaf.)*

The kidney/bladder stretch

Touch Therapies

Massage

Standing for too long damages the bladder and kidney meridian, which can cause fatigue and low backaches. Traditionally, Bladder 23 is one of the best points to aid tiredness related to the kidney region (*see Figure, page 124*). Make the kidney sound 'WOOOOOO' and visualize a dark blue colour as you rub these points on either side of your spine at around waist height.

Reflexology

The bladder reflex point is on the inside of both feet near the heel. Trace up the tendon, which is the reflex zone for the urethra until you reach the kidney point. Gently massage this area by 'walking' your thumb from the bladder to the kidney, feeling for any 'crystals'. (*See page 30 for massage techniques.*)

Reflexology points for the bladder (shaded)

Acupressure

Acupressure is widely used to improve and maintain kidney and bladder function; used on a regular basis it can be very supportive to these organs. Although the bladder may appear to have a relatively simple task, the points on its meridian relate to every organ and part of the body and have an influence over all the other meridians. The areas covered by this meridian are the neck, shoulders, back, buttocks, back of the thighs and the fleshy part of the calves.

Bladder 1 is located at the inner corner of both eyes; it rises vertically over the forehead and down the back of the neck to the upper back, where it splits into two parallel lines: one 2.5 cm away from the spine and the other 5 cm away. These parallel lines then run down the back, through the kidneys and bladder at the lumbar region of the back, then down the back of the thigh where the two lines join behind the knee. The meridian then continues as one channel along the back of the calf and down the outside of the foot to finish at the outer nailbed of the smallest toe.

It is very therapeutic to stimulate the part of the bladder meridian that runs down the back. This can be done by a partner massaging up and down the channels, noting where the tension knots lie. Alternatively, you could tie two tennis balls into a sock, lie on your back with the balls 2.5–5 cm away from either side of the spine and gently roll the balls up and down vertically over a small section of your back.

The bladder meridian

123   *The Bladder*

Bladder 23 acupressure point

BLADDER 23

A major point to strengthen the kidney and bladder and boost
energy levels. Place your thumbs on either side of your waist and
use your middle fingers to find the point, which is on both sides
of the spine. Alternatively, rub the back of your clenched fist over
this area, gently tapping it to stimulate the region.

Essential Oils

Bergamot: a powerful disinfectant of the urinary system.
   Valuable for inflammation and infection. Assists and prevents
   infections such as urethritis from spreading to the bladder.
   Must never be used on the skin when in strong sunlight, as it
   is phototoxic. *Strength factor: Medium*

Cedarwood: useful for genito-urinary infections triggered by either cold or damp conditions. A mild diuretic, can also soothe and relieve the pain and discomfort that so often accompanies cystitis. Bestows extra resistance and strength during times of crisis and is a useful 'grounding' oil, helpful as an aid to meditation. *Strength factor: Weak*

Geranium: one of the best oils for the tendency towards armouring that is representative of a bladder imbalance. Lets emotional sensitivity in, gently dissolving the barriers we sometimes put up around ourselves and helping us to develop softness and receptivity, while still affording protection to our vulnerable inner self. An anti-inflammatory oil, useful for cystitis, and a diuretic, stimulating the elimination of excess fluid. *Strength factor: Strong*

Juniper: one of the strongest diuretic oils available. Purifies and detoxifies. Has anti-infectious properties, ideal for cleansing the body and treating cystitis and urinary tract infections. Prolonged use, however, can over-stimulate the kidneys: use only in moderation and for short periods. Provides emotional strength, support and confidence to those who have isolated themselves due to psychological fears and insecurities. *Strength factor: Medium*

Sandalwood: a very powerful urinary antiseptic, yet mild and gentle on the system. Alleviates the discomfort caused by cystitis of a hot and inflammatory nature. Comforting and sedative on an emotional level. *Strength factor: Weak*

Chamomile, Pine, Parsley and Garlic oils can also be used to treat urethritis and cystitis; Tea Tree, Myrrh and Lavender help to clear fungal infections which may also be prevalent.

Emotions

'Armouring' is a key emotion linked to the bladder and this can manifest on many different levels, with the resulting tension corresponding to different layers of muscle. Major surface muscles of the back include the trapezius, latissimus dorsi and the gluteus maximus; important deep muscles include the spinalis and sacrospinalis. Tension in these muscles is very common and is also associated with great emotional strain.

The bladder, like the kidneys, is affected by fear. A person prone to deep depression and an inability to cope with life situations or change may have an energy imbalance in the bladder. This is particularly true of children, where insecurities and anxiety can lead to bedwetting. In adults, however, bladder disorders are sometimes linked to feelings of suspicion or jealousy over extended periods of time.

Flower Remedies

Rockwater: the Bach flower remedy for those who are over-rigid and strict in their approach to life, often becoming so hard on themselves that they do not experience even the simplest pleasures in life and ignore their inner needs, resulting in rigidity in the body and muscles, especially those running up either side of the spine. Can bring out qualities such as softness and the ability to be more adaptable and flexible in life.

Vine: for those who are very inflexible and self-opinionated, domineering and possess a will of iron. These traits can lead to extreme stiffness in the body, especially in the back, where the bladder meridian pathway runs. Vine allows such personality types to excel and make the most of their natural leadership qualities, but will help to soften their rigid nature.

You may also find some appropriate flower remedies for supporting the Water element in the chapter on the kidney (page 142).

Affirmations

- My bladder releases all fluid wastes.
- I am adaptable and feel able to open myself to the flow of life.
- I absorb a dark blue healing light, and feel it cleansing and soothing my bladder.
- I am fearless.

See also the kidneys chapter, page 129, for affirmations that may be used in conjunction with these.

Meditation for the Water Element

Before beginning this meditation, familiarize yourself with the diagrams of the relevant meridians (i.e. for the bladder and kidneys). Remember that *qi* is pronounced 'chee', and that all meridians are bilateral (running along both sides of the body); for the purposes of this meditation the meridian points on only one side of the body are focused on. If possible, tape this meditation, reading it out clearly and slowly in a soft tone of voice.

Find a peaceful place to relax and unwind. Close your eyes. Focus your attention on your breathing and, as you begin to notice it deepening, gently let any thoughts that come into your mind float by like clouds in the sky. For a few minutes, practise the breathing exercise recommended in the Lung chapter (*page 183*).

Water Meditation

Imagine yourself sitting comfortably in a large, old armchair in a room which is lit only by the warm light of a fire. The brilliant embers glow from orange to red and the flickering flames create magical patterns. Outside it is a cold, crisp Winter's evening and bare branches of the trees with their covering of snow are outlined against dark indigo skies. The ground is frozen and hard and all is still and silent. Take your eyes back with relief to the fire and focus on the pictures of mysterious caverns, inviting exploration and leading into the light. See this as a time of drawing in and consolidating your energy; a time where any dark fears or anxieties can be transmuted into feelings of hope and expectation of the bright future to come with the Spring. Consciously take the deep warmth and glow from the fire and imagine that you can fill your lower back and stomach with this warmth. Feel it spreading and flowing into your kidneys. Intensify the warmth and know that it is supporting and regenerating your kidney *qi*. Allow this warmth to flow down to your knees and feet; feel the deep radiance that this energy brings.

Now focus your energy on the base of your foot where the Kidney meridian begins. Begin to build and intensify the *qi* at Kidney 1 on the sole of your foot. Send the *qi* up the inner part of your leg to your navel, where you can concentrate it and sense it filling the whole area, including your kidneys, with warmth and healing energy. Then allow the *qi* to travel to a point just beneath your collar bone, where the meridian ends. Take this energy next to the inner corner of your eye, which is the start of the Bladder meridian. Feel the *qi* flowing across the top of your head and down the back of your neck, then see it divide into two parallel channels that run down either side of your spine. Imagine that the healing energy clears any obstruction or rigidity held in your back. Allow the *qi* to continue along the meridian pathways down the back of your legs, through your knees and down until the end of the meridian at your little toes.

Sense your energy becoming stronger, then begin to move your fingers and toes, feeling yourself rejuvenated and regenerated ... and, in your own time, open your eyes and stretch your body out.

The Kidneys

 The kidneys are a pair of ear-shaped organs located above the waist, towards the back of the body.

Western Function

The main function of the kidneys according to Western physiology is to filter blood and body fluids. A large portion of the body's wastes are eliminated through the kidneys, as they help to remove poisons from the liver. High levels of toxins in the body put the kidneys under pressure.

According to Western medicine, severe imbalances in the kidneys can cause cystitis and other bladder disorders and even prostate disorders in men. If the kidneys cannot purify the body when toxic waste levels are too high, calcium and other by-products may be deposited in the kidneys and other vital organs, possibly contributing to arterial sclerosis, cell degeneration and kidney stones. It is also thought that kidney stones can develop when the moisture level in the body is too low; this is one of the reasons why it is recommended that everyone should drink several glasses of pure water every day.

The heart and kidneys have a close relationship, as blood and waste is separated and the purified blood returns to the heart to be circulated around the body. Approximately 5 litres per hour of blood flow through the kidneys, to be broken down into nutritional components. Too much salt in the diet can contribute to high blood pressure, as the kidneys adjust blood pressure.

The kidneys are connected to the adrenal glands, which sit on top of each kidney (ad-renal being the medical term for kidney-related), and to adrenaline, a hormone released at critical and stressful times. With allergies on the increase, coupled with stress in our daily lives, the kidneys and adrenals are often overworked, giving rise to a wide range of symptoms including fatigue.

Traditional Chinese Interpretation

Element:	Water
Partner organ:	Bladder
Climate:	Cold
Season:	Winter
Colour:	Blue/black
Time of day:	5–7 p.m.
Body tissue:	Bones and marrow
Voice sound:	Moaning
Sense organ:	Ears
Reflector:	Head hair
Taste:	Salty
Emotion:	Fear

SYMPTOMS OF IMBALANCE

Emotional
Fear • Wishy-washy behaviour • Lack of willpower • Panic attacks • Weakness, timidity • Apprehension • Learning difficulties • Feeling overwhelmed • Fear of failure • Paranoid, suspicious behaviour • Complaining • Depression

---

Physical
Premature ageing and senility • Sterility and impotence • Poor sexual development • Retarded growth • Dark bags under the eyes • Craving for salty foods • Broken, split, dull hair • Oedema (fluid-retention) and bloating • Lower back pain • Premature greying of hair, loss of hair • Soft or brittle, weak bones • Urination problems • Aversion to cold • Lethargy, frequent yawning • Knee problems •

The Chinese believe that it is essential that we preserve our kidneys, the deepest organ in the body storing our *Jing. Jing* is thought to determine our constitutional make-up and govern our development, especially in the early stages of life. *Jing* is also thought to be difficult to replenish once it is depleted. *Jing* is called the 'root of life' because it is the source of reproduction, development and maturation; cases of sterility and impotence, or slow sexual maturation are kidney problems. The kidneys store reproductive energy and are very important in determining the length of our lives and our level of vitality. All sexual energy comes from the kidneys, so any sexual or reproductive dysfunction (such as impotence, frigidity or sterility) can be traced to the kidneys. Premature ageing, lethargy, lack of perception, wishy-washy behaviour and aching in the lower part of the back also reflect a lack of vital *Jing*. The entire body and all its organs need this extremely precious, inherited essence in order to thrive and survive.

In Chinese medicine, the kidneys and adrenal glands are believed to contribute to the warmth of the body, our energy levels, sexual appetite, and strength in general.

Long hours working or studying can weaken the kidneys and can have a negative impact on the spleen. The body doesn't lie and the effects of tobacco, alcohol, eating on the run and lack of exercise will eventually catch up with you and impair your health!

As mentioned, the kidneys are strongly related to sexual performance. Too much sex and frequent pregnancies can weaken the body and drain the kidney energy, thus reducing our vitality. The Chinese used to regard sex as a cause of disease; a book entitled *The Classic of the Simple Girl* (Sui Dynasty, AD 581–618) made the following recommendations on the frequency of male ejaculation.

Male Sexual Health

Age	Average Health	Above Average Health
20	Once a day	Twice a day
30	Every other day	Once a day
40	Every 4 days	Every 3 days
50	Every 10 days	Every 5 days
60	Every 20 days	Every 10 days
70+	Abstain!	Once a month

Ejaculation for a man and, to a lesser extent, orgasm for a woman deplete the kidney essence.

Apart from the kidneys, the liver and heart notably contribute to a normal and happy sexual life. As the heart is also related to the kidneys, the two must support and nourish each other. Just as a kidney deficiency can weaken the heart, a heart deficiency caused by sadness and anxiety can weaken the kidneys and cause impotence or the inability to reach orgasm. The liver is responsible for the smooth flow of blood and *qi*, particularly in the lower part of the body. Stagnation here can influence our sex life and lead to inability to reach orgasm or frigidity/impotence.

Our kidney essence is known to be depleted by the ageing process. Common symptoms in old age such as hearing difficulties, brittle bones and memory problems arise as a result of the decline of kidney essence.

SELF-HELP FOR KEEPING YOUR KIDNEYS HEALTHY

Chinese Nutrition

Foods for the Water Element

Grain: beans and peas	Fruit: dates
Meat: pork	Vegetable: sea vegetables

The taste of the Water element (which encompasses the kidneys and the bladder) is salty, so small amounts of naturally salty foods in the diet are beneficial. However, excessive cravings for salt, or a dislike of salt, means you should keep an eye on the health of the kidneys. The salty flavour enters the kidneys and in small amounts can either nourish and support them or in excessive amounts can aggravate a Water imbalance.

The kidneys regulate the acid balance in the body and the mineral levels in the blood. All kidney problems are thought to have a strong link with acid/alkaline imbalances in the body. Ideally our acid/alkaline balance should be 80 per cent alkaline and 20 per cent acid, although in modern-day living the reverse is often true.

Dietary Tips

1. Celery is high in organic sodium; miso (a Japanese fermented rice puree) contains salt and the lactobacteria that are so important to our health to restore the pH balance in the intestines.
2. Tamari sauce – the wheat-free version of soy sauce – is a good substitute for salt, to be used in moderation in cooking. If you do consume salt, ensure that it is sea salt.
3. Fish is also considered to be highly beneficial for the kidneys, perhaps because of seafood's connection with water! Oysters

are particularly rich in zinc, a mineral that supports the reproductive system and have a well-earned reputation as an aphrodisiac!

4. Aduki, black and kidney beans are rich in potassium and have a special affinity with the kidneys, possibly due to their kidney-like colour and shape.

5. Grains such as buckwheat, rice, barley and millet. Millet is alkaline and can help lower acid levels in the body. Buckwheat has warming properties and is known to heat the blood and the whole body. Wheat and rye are the most acidic of all grains and so are best avoided while you are working on raising the alkaline levels in your body.

6. Beetroot is a very cleansing food for the kidneys and is high in potassium, magnesium and vitamin A.

7. Wintertime is the best time of the year to eat meat and the Chinese recommend that foods such as bone marrow, oxtail, kidneys and red meat are added to stews. However, with the current scare over some of these foods, always search out a reputable organic farmer to ensure that the meat is safe, and free from additives and steroids.

8. When in season, fruits of the forest such as blackberries and cranberries are excellent cleansers (note that strawberries and raspberries are exceptions to this).

9. Black sesame seeds are thought to improve the quality of the blood, return grey hair to its original colour, build muscles, sharpen vision, lubricate the body (thus promoting semen and marrow production), strengthen bones and, consumed on a regular basis, to be an excellent preventative tonic which will help you to retain your youthfulness.

10. Other foods to increase in your diet are walnuts, all leafy green vegetables (such as broccoli, watercress, parsley), green beans and peas, courgettes, lettuce, celery, various forms of green cabbage (such as Savoy, wintergreen), beetroot, swedes, turnips and marrows.

11. Sea vegetables are essential to include in the diet and they are easy to assimilate as the protein is almost predigested and, coming from the sea, they have a real affinity with the Water element. They are extremely high in minerals, and can be added to dishes to increase the nutritional value. Kombu can

be put into soups and stews; adding a piece of kombu to the water and cider vinegar you soak beans and pulses in reduces the flatulence that some legumes can bestow! Wakame (tiny strips of seaweed) can be soaked for 10 minutes in water, drained and then added to a stir-fry with rice. If you use a small amount to start with, you really cannot taste it (for those who are repulsed by the thought of eating seaweed!) but will get all those valuable minerals from including it in your diet.

12. Reduce the amount of acid-forming foods in your diet such as coffee, tea and refined foods such as pastry, bread, biscuits, sweets and other convenience foods.

13. The nightshade family (peppers, aubergines, tomatoes and potatoes) together with dairy products, shellfish, citrus fruits and nuts are thought to raise levels of a protein by-product called albumen, which can promote congestion in the kidneys.

14. Increase alkaline-rich foods such as fresh fruit and vegetables and millet. Water-rich fruits such as water melons and grapes are said to help prevent kidney stones (although if you suffer from feeling the cold, consume them only in warmer months); celery, asparagus and kelp all stimulate urination.

When the moisture level in the body falls too low, kidney stones can develop, and this is one of the reasons why it is important to drink pure water every day (not coffee or even herbal teas, but pure water). Although the current thinking is to drink copious amounts of water, the kidneys can only move six glasses of water a day (this includes liquids that are already in the body as well as what you drink), so it is important to balance the amount of fluid you consume: too much can be as bad as too little. Also, iced water is not advisable – keep it room temperature or even warmer during the Winter months.

Helpful herbs and spices
• Cinnamon has a particular affinity for the kidney and is an excellent spice to include in your diet. It can be added to foods, or a hot tea can be made by boiling fresh cinnamon bark for about 20 minutes. Cinnamon is also found in some herbal teas. Other useful warming spices include ginger and fenugreek.

- Roasted chicory is a coffee substitute that centres the body and encourages the *qi* to move downwards.
- Nettles are supportive to the adrenal glands and can help to remove stones from the kidneys. Try in the form of nettle tea.
- Rehmannia is a key herb used in traditional Chinese medicine to tone the kidney when it is '*yin*-deficient'.

Exercise

According to Chinese medicine, Winter is the worst time of the year for strenuous exercise; instead it is a time for conserving and replenishing energy levels. Enough exercise to get the circulation moving and to warm the body up is ideal during this season. Brisk walking and a swimming programme are suitable, as light exercises such as these are the best ways to get warm and ensure that the *qi* and blood keep moving throughout the body. T'ai Chi and Qigong are particularly good forms of exercise as they do not deplete the body of vital *qi*.

The stretch for the kidney and bladder meridian is described on page 120.

Touch Therapies

Massage

Traditionally, the meridian point known as Bladder 23 can be rubbed to stimulate the kidney region; Kidney 27 should be held as you make the sound 'WOOOOOO' and visualize a dark blue colour (*see figure of Bladder 23, page 124, and the Kidney meridian, overleaf*).

Reflexology

The kidney reflex cannot be separated from those of the bladder and ureter. The bladder reflexology point is located on the inside of both feet near the heel. Trace up the tendon, which represents the urethra, until you reach the kidney reflex. Gently massage this area by 'walking' your thumb from the bladder to the kidney, feeling for any 'crystals'. (*See page 30 for massage techniques.*)

Reflexology points for the kidneys (shaded)

Acupressure

The kidney meridian actually begins on the sole of the foot and travels up the inside ankle to the inner thigh. It then goes within and connects to both the kidney and bladder before running back to the surface where it travels up the front of the body and finishes at the base of the collar bone – Kidney 27 *(see diagram overleaf).*

kidney 27

kidney 1

The kidney meridian and acupuncture points

KIDNEY 3

Kidney 3 is located on the inside of the ankle, halfway between the Achilles tendon and the ankle bone. This point enhances the energy of the kidneys and also can help to strengthen willpower, thus restoring both courage and self-confidence.

KIDNEY 6

Kidney 6 is located near Kidney 3 and is one finger-width directly beneath the inside of the ankle bone in a little hollow. It can be sensitive to pressure, so apply it with care. This point helps to balance the Water element and the emotions that correspond to it (such as fear and depression). It also supports the lungs by opening the chest and can calm the mind. For both Kidney 3 and Kidney 6, hold your heel with one hand and gently stimulate the acupressure point by rubbing it with the thumb of your other hand in a circular motion. Do be gentle with this area and never use too much pressure.

Kidney 3 (under the right thumb) and 6 (above) acupressure points

These two points along with Bladder 23 would greatly benefit from moxibustion when there are symptoms of fatigue, weakness and cold.

It is important to protect the kidney area. The Japanese used to do this by wearing a *harikame* – a band worn around the hara area to support the immune system and keep the body healthy and strong. You can make your own version by tying a scarf around your waist. Ensure that the scarf is approximately 16 cm wide at the back, and covers you 8 cm above and below the waist. It will also keep you very warm in bed, allowing you to wake feeling more refreshed and rested.

Essential Oils

Cedarwood: strengthens the energy of the kidneys; has an affinity for the genito-urinary system, good for bladder infections. Gives extra strength on an emotional level during difficult times, helping to transform these periods into opportunities to learn and gain spiritual insight and wisdom. *Strength factor: Weak*

Cypress: detoxifies and decongests the body, helping to restore balance and equilibrium to the acid/alkali levels. Helps with hidden fears or fears of unknown origin. Added to the bath (4–6 drops along with the same amount of the Bach flower remedy Aspen), it can soothe away such fears. Also helpful for depression associated with being oppressed by another. *Strength factor: Medium*

Fennel: has an affinity for the kidneys and, by strengthening the kidney *yang* energy, plays a supportive role to the spleen. *Strength factor: Strong*

Geranium: helps on an emotional level to balance willpower when we feel unable to contain and control our personal ambition to succeed. Helps to bring out the qualities needed to soften and slow this driving force. Gently supports energy and calms the mind. Excellent for hormonal imbalance and lymphatic congestion. *Strength factor: Strong*

Ginger: strengthens energy and fire, helping to activate willpower when we are apathetic or procrastinating; stimulates inspiration and creativity. Can help to rekindle the flames of passion when they have been dampened by an imbalance in the Water element! *Strength factor: Medium*

Juniper: an excellent diuretic, helping to flush out excess water from the system. A decongestant, eliminating toxins and stimulating the lymphatic system. Helps to combat infections, especially in the genito-urinary system. A warming and stimulating oil that warms cold hands and lifts fatigue. Uplifts and inspires those who have allowed negativity and fear to consume their thoughts and control their actions. Drives away the fear of failure connected to self-doubt and insecurity, restoring resolve and determination. *Strength factor: Medium*

Thyme: adds warmth to the kidneys and helps us to overcome fears that arise from a known cause. Instils courage and boosts low morale by replacing poor self-esteem and apathy with vigour, confidence and drive. *Strength factor: Strong*

Rosemary: raises low self-esteem and encourages optimism and confidence. A supreme memory stimulant. *Strength factor: Strong*

NB All essential oils should be used with care and true kidney ailments need prompt medical attention and proper diagnosis.

Emotions

The kidneys are known as the seat of fear, which we can see manifested when adrenaline is released in 'fight or flight' situations. When the kidneys are weakened or damaged, this may indicate that unexpressed or unacknowledged fears are building up within us. Kidney problems can therefore be related to holding on to old emotional patterns, or to negative emotions that are not being consciously released. Shock too is associated with the kidneys – this is said to explain the peculiar occurrence of people who can go grey overnight, or develop a white streak in their hair after hearing shocking news.

Willpower and ambition are governed by the Water element. Anyone lacking willpower is expressing a symptom of a Water imbalance. However, if the energy in the kidneys is excessive, workaholism may result, as we can be driven on by a fear of failure.

Metaphysically, kidney stones have been seen as the manifestation of unshed tears or sadness. Releasing these feelings indicates a movement forward to a new state of being.

Fully grounding the body is important to strengthen the base and kidney energy. 'Grounding' activities include any work with the earth such as gardening, walking in the countryside, etc. Lean up against a tree and feel the strength and power it gives to you. Imagine that roots are coming out of your toes; see these roots going deep into the earth, anchoring you firmly to the ground. Feel safe and secure and allow your fears to be absorbed by the Earth and transmuted (*see Earth meditation, page 62*).

Flower Remedies

Aspen: for vague fears and apprehensions and unconscious fears when you cannot understand where the feelings are coming from. Often people who need Aspen are sensitive to psychic influences – children who need the light on at night because they are scared of ghosts benefit from Aspen. A glass of water with 2–4 drops of this remedy left beside the bed at night will help children who wake with nightmares.

Mimulus: for tangible fears that arise in everyday life. Those who need Mimulus are often sensitive souls with a delicate constitution, which ties in with the kidney type of personality, who has to be careful not to burn the candle at both ends.

Olive: Exhaustion is felt both mentally and physically when our kidney *qi* is depleted. Olive restores strength and vitality to body and soul.

Rock Rose: the remedy for extreme, acute fears that border on terror. For those almost frozen into a state of fear; children who wake screaming after a particularly bad nightmare should be given this remedy in the same way as Aspen.

Star of Bethlehem: the remedy for trauma and shock, which have a profound affect on the state of the kidneys. Soothes and comforts, restoring the body's self-healing mechanism and heralding the return of calm.

You may also find some appropriate flower remedies for supporting the Water element in the chapter on the bladder (page 126).

Affirmations

- My kidneys cleanse and care for my body.
- I allow the *qi* to regenerate in my kidneys, replenishing the very core of my being.
- I am safe and secure and able to face any challenges that may arise.
- My willpower is resolute and gives me newfound strength.
- I cherish my kidneys as they are the root of all life and new beginnings.

See also the Bladder chapter, page 115, for affirmations that may be used in conjunction with these.

Meditation for the Water Element
See Bladder chapter, page 127.

The Wood Element

Partner Organs: Liver and gallbladder, which have a very close relationship not only in the Chinese system, but also in Western medicine. For example, the liver as seen in Western pathology produces bile, which is then stored and concentrated in the gallbladder.

Climate: Wind. It is essential to protect your body from the wind, the most vulnerable area being the back of the neck and shoulders. Springtime colds and flus can be greatly reduced by following the simple advice of wearing a scarf. The liver is also susceptible to *internal wind* in the body (not flatulence!), which can give rise to stiffness, numbness, convulsions, twitches, pains that move in the body and clumsiness.

Season: The Wood element is linked to Spring, the time of year when the earth begins to burst alive with energy and new growth. The growth of plants can mirror how the body energy changes with the seasons. The body's energy rises and moves from within to the surface in Spring; plants, too, begin to grow above the ground, their growth upward and outward.

Colour: Green is the colour of the Wood element – interestingly the colour associated with jealousy and revenge, the emotions linked to the gallbladder. An obsession with or an aversion to this colour can point to an imbalance in the Wood element. Chinese practitioners with a trained eye will notice a green tinge on the face, a viable diagnostic indication of imbalance.

Time of Day: The time the gallbladder is in power, according to the Chinese body clock, is 11 p.m.–1 a.m. The liver follows on from 1–3 a.m. Failing to sleep, or waking between these times, can point to an imbalance in the liver or gallbladder. This element also has an influence on the quality and length of sleep, and can induce dreams of trials, fights and suicide according to ancient Chinese texts. It is important to be in bed before this element comes into power as the liver is involved in filtering the blood. To do this effectively, the body needs to be horizontal because when you are up and about, the liver directs blood to the parts of the body needing it. If, for example, you are exercising, the blood is sent to nourish the muscles. Ideally you should aim to be in bed before 11 p.m., otherwise the liver energy is diverted from its important physical function of cleaning and renewing the blood. Waking unrefreshed and tired in the morning can show that the liver hasn't purified the blood efficiently. Excess artificial light, working for long hours or shift work through the night can also prevent the liver from regenerating effectively.

Body Tissue: The Wood element controls the tendons and ligaments and the way in which these interact with the muscles. If the liver has not cleansed the blood sufficiently or if there is a deficiency of blood, the tendons will suffer from malnutrition – giving rise to stiffness, difficulty flexing and extending the joints, numbness and spasms. Therefore, for any diseases that involve the tendons we must look at the Wood element.

Voice Sound: Shouting – a very obvious connection as the emotion of the liver, anger, frequently manifests as emotional outbursts and raging arguments as the pressure cooker lid finally blows off! Someone with a loud voice is also demonstrating 'liverish' tendencies.

Sense Organ: The Wood element nourishes the eyes (with the gallbladder). The health of the eyes is seen as being dependent on the health of the liver, so any visual disturbances can be interpreted as a reflection of the state of your liver. If a problem occurs in the liver, the eyes can suffer from dryness, redness, night blindness, 'floaters' (black spots before the eyes), cataracts, glaucoma or blurred vision.

Reflector: The nails are considered an extension of the tendons, so problems such as changes in nail colour, brittle nails, ridges on the nails or weak, splitting nails all tell us that something about the Wood element is being imbalanced.

Symptoms of Imbalance: The liver is the key organ associated with the Wood element. A healthy liver is like a tender young tree that is green and flexible, yet firmly rooted into the earth. The sap is fresh and vital like the blood in our body when it is clean and pure. As it bends in the wind, its movements are graceful and fluid, just like our body when in balance, with energy flowing smoothly and effortlessly. When the liver energy stagnates, however, we can become brittle, wooden and inflexible in both body and mind.

The Gallbladder

 The gallbladder is a pear-shaped organ the size of your thumb, situated underneath the liver.

Western Function

The gallbladder cooperates with the liver, which makes about 2 litres a day of a liquid called bile which is concentrated and stored in the gallbladder. Bile acts like a washing-up powder, breaking up fats in the food.

When food enters the small intestine, a hormone is released which instructs the gallbladder to contract and send bile directly to the small intestine to assist in breaking down fatty foods. Salts in the bile help the body absorb fat-soluble vitamins. Synthetic drugs, together with natural hormones and steroids, are excreted in the bile. The bile is then sent back to the liver to be recycled, and so the process turns full circle. Bile is, in addition, a good laxative which ensures that peristalsis (movement of the large intestines) takes place.

Gallstones affect about 15 per cent of the population. They form when cholesterol levels rise. Steroids and the contraceptive pill predispose us to gallstones, so does too much fat and protein in the diet – ironically, too little fat and skipping meals are also contributory factors. Eating a meal which contains a little fat, preferably olive oil, will stimulate the gallbladder into releasing bile. Low bile levels can result in an overgrowth of bacteria in the small intestine, leading to fermentation of the foods and bloating.

Traditional Chinese Interpretation

Element:	Wood
Partner organ:	Liver
Climate:	Wind
Season:	Spring
Colour:	Green
Time of day:	11 p.m.–1 a.m.
Body tissue:	Tendons/ligaments
Voice sound:	Shouting
Sense organ:	Eyes
Reflector:	Nails
Taste:	Sour
Emotion:	Anger

SYMPTOMS OF IMBALANCE

Emotional
Jealousy • Resentment • Aggressive behaviour • Indecision • Frustration • Unexpressed anger • Bitterness

Physical
Pain on right side of trunk • Migraines and headaches • Stiff shoulders and neck area • Weak, splitting nails • Difficulty

---

In Chinese medicine the gallbladder and liver are affected by anger, frustration and bottled-up resentment. We all know expressions such as 'she had the gall to accuse me' and other references to people being 'liverish'. Irritability, thirst, headaches and a bitter taste in the mouth can point to gallbladder trouble. Stagnation of energy in the body can harm the spleen, and symptoms of imbalance such as oedema and lethargy may become apparent. Excess damp in the body leads it to try to create more heat, bringing another set of problems known as 'damp heat'. This often occurs in the pelvis; vaginal infections, thrush, fibroids and other genital problems can manifest as a result.

SELF-HELP FOR KEEPING YOUR GALLBLADDER HEALTHY

Chinese Nutrition

Foods for the Wood Element

Grain: wheat	Fruit: peach
Meat: chicken	Vegetable: leek

The taste for the Wood element is sour, so craving a lot of sour foods, e.g. lemons, sauerkraut and pickled snacks, can be feeding a Wood imbalance, or an indication that the body is trying to correct one. The body knows what it needs to strengthen itself.

Certain foods have a negative effect on the gallbladder – in particular very greasy foods, cholesterol and excessive amounts of alcohol. However, a small quantity of alcohol (half a glass of wine or beer) can increase the breakdown of cholesterol, making less of it available to produce gallstones. In Greece, where olive oil is consumed regularly, gallstones are relatively unknown. Vegetarians too have fewer gallstones than the average, probably due to the higher levels of vitamin C and fibre in their diets.

Fasting or even skipping a meal (particularly breakfast) can bring on gallstones, as can following a low fat diet. The body needs at least 5 to 10 grams of fat in one meal each day to stimulate the gallbladder to release bile. When fat intake is drastically cut, the gallbladder does not contract to expel bile as often, so it can build up, possibly triggering the formation of gallstones. Increasing the vegetable protein and fibre in your diet helps offset this. Eating smaller and more frequent meals – little and often – helps to prevent a concentration of bile in the gallbladder.

Dietary Tips

1. Foods that are supportive to the gallbladder include artichokes, green beans, beetroot and greens, carrots, dandelions, endive, fennel, lemon, kale, mustard greens, nettles, olive oil, parsley, radish, sweet potato and watercress.
2. Soya bean protein (organic), nuts, beans, lentils, peas and lima beans help prevent gallstones.
3. Supplement your diet with lecithin – a well-known fat emulsifier which helps to keep cholesterol in solution.
4. Try cooking using turmeric, an Indian spice that is excellent for the liver and gallbladder. See the chapter on the liver (*page 168*) for additional herbs and spices to aid the Wood element.
5. The B-complex vitamins (found in whole grain foods) help the gallbladder to empty more efficiently.

See the chapter on the liver, page 163, for further information about foods for the Wood element.

Exercise

Exercise that helps us to release stored-up frustrations and tensions also helps to reduce stagnation in the liver and gallbladder. Do ensure, however, that exercise does not become excessive or depleting. Gentle movement and stretching exercises such as T'ai Chi and yoga encourage flexibility (important for the Wood element as it is prone to tension and stiffness). If you feel rigor mortis setting in, loosen up those muscles by simply swinging your arms and legs gently to improve circulation.

The stretch for the gallbladder and liver meridians involves sitting on the floor with your legs as wide apart as possible.

Ensure that your back is straight. Put your hands together, stretch your arms over your head and take a deep breath. Exhale slowly as you stretch forward gently towards your right foot or calf – aim to reach for your toes. Go as far as your body can manage, never over-stretch. Instead, relax into a comfortable stretch and take some deep breaths. Visualize a white light flowing into the meridians and your muscles; see the congestion melting away. You should feel the stretch along the outside of your right leg and the inside of your left. Repeat twice then slowly bring your body back into an upright position. Repeat on the left side. Remember that it may take many weeks or months to achieve this. Always work at your own pace and ensure that you have warmed the muscles in your body for 10 minutes prior to stretching. If possible, join a local yoga class where you can be guided and personally instructed.

The gallbladder/liver stretch

Touch Therapies

Reflexology

The reflex point for the gallbladder is situated on the right foot, just beneath the liver reflex. Gently massage by walking your thumb over this area, feeling for any hard, granular lumps. Finish by massaging the foot with a base oil to which some essential oils have been added. (*See page 30 for massage techniques.*)

Reflexology point for the gallbladder (shaded)

Massage

Regular massage is ideal to soften stiff muscles. As the Wood element is responsible for the smooth flow of *qi* in the body, soothing an imbalance will focus on easing inner tension and frustration. If this tension accumulates and goes inward, then depression can result which will benefit from specific oils that help to break up stagnant emotions such as unexpressed anger or resentment (*see Essential Oils, page 157*).

Acupressure

The gallbladder meridian (*see page 156*) is the longest in the body. Its pathway begins at the outer corner of either eye and zigzags around the head, running down the back of the head and neck into the shoulders, round the rib cage, into the buttocks, and down the outside of the leg, finishing at the nail of the fourth toe.

GALLBLADDER 20

This is at the back of the head, located between the base of the skull and the neck muscles in a little hollow of the spinal column. This point has an impact on the entire body and can relieve tension in the head and improve circulation to the face and eyes. It can release neck and head tension and will often be sensitive to the touch if there is congestion in these areas. Helps with dizziness and insomnia; can soothe and calm the nerves (*see page 158*).

GALLBLADDER 21

This point is found at the top of the shoulders, located on the big muscle at the base of the neck. It is easy to find as the point is often very tight and sore! This is a classic point for reflecting our state of tension and disharmony. Massaging it eases stiffness in the neck and can also relieve pain in the shoulders and upper back.

These two points have traditionally been used to release headaches, ease fatigue and help with nervous disorders; they also have a connection with the sexual organs (so do not work on either point if you are pregnant).

The gallbladder meridian

156   *Body Wisdom*

Gallbladder 20 (under thumbs) and 21 (on shoulders) acupressure points

Essential Oils

Bergamot: regulates and smoothes liver *qi*, encouraging an even flow of energy around the body. Calms and regulates the nervous system, nervous tension often being created by *qi* stagnation. Alleviates and releases bottled-up resentment and frustration. *Strength factor: Medium*

Bitter orange: unblocks stagnant *qi* in the liver, gallbladder, stomach and intestines. Helps with emotional tension, insomnia and nauseous headaches or migraines. Ideal for abdominal distension and flatulence, indigestion, nausea, vomiting and constipation. Stimulates the gallbladder and encourages the flow of bile. *Strength factor: Medium*

Chamomile: eases resentment, frustration and depression that result from energy stagnating in the Wood element. Has an impact on the solar plexus (our nerve centre) so is extremely helpful for nervous tension of either mental and physical origin. *Strength factor: Strong*

Lavender: cools and calms, taking the heat out of unexpressed anger that can manifest as inner rage, frustration, resentment and general irritability. Encourages the movement and flow of *qi*, releasing pent-up energy. *Strength factor: Weak*

Other oils of benefit include Peppermint and Rosemary.

Emotions

In Chinese medicine the gallbladder and liver are affected by anger, frustration and bottled-up resentment. These feelings deplete our energy levels and can lead to long-term health problems.

The Chinese believe anger in short explosive bursts is actually healthy, but in our society, especially for women, this is often deemed unacceptable. Seeing a counsellor or even talking to a close friend to get feelings out and free the body of emotional pain must be a priority. Try releasing pent-up emotions by punching the air or a pillow, or do what the Native American tribespeople do: the 'power stomp'. If you have a drum, play the drum too! Shake your hands to release any stress held within as if you were shaking it out of your body. Punch the air to get it all out. Stamp your feet and make the sound 'Ho', allowing it to come from deep within, not just your throat. If you are angry with someone or something, let your feelings out in this safe way, rather than keeping them inside bubbling away until you finally explode!

The Chinese believe that when the gallbladder is working efficiently, its owner will be able to take clear and decisive action. They have an expression for this: 'Big Gallbladder' (meaning courageous). When the Wood element is healthy, we are graceful and flexible both physically and mentally. Our powers of judgement and decision-making are sound, our vision clear and our actions resolute.

Flower Remedies

Beech: for a tense, stiff body and a critical, irritable, dissatisfied mind. Loosens and relaxes the rigidity that encompasses both mind and body and fosters tolerance and compassion.

Holly: for aggressive emotions such as jealousy, envy, frustration and pent-up anger as well as outright rage, hatred and distrust which we find difficult to hold inside. Helps to transmute these emotions into their opposite: compassion and love.

Scleranthus: for indecision, affording clarity and allowing for decisive action to be taken. Helps with restlessness, fluctuating moods and changeable symptoms – physical and emotional ones. Focuses the mind and restores harmony and inner balance.

Wild Oat: helps to give direction and a sense of purpose at times when we feel vague and undecided.

Willow: for resentment and bitterness; for those who bear a grudge and blame others rather than accepting personal responsibility. Helps us to accept our negative emotions and take responsibility for our actions. Encourages faith, calm and optimism.

You will also find some appropriate flower remedies for supporting the Wood element in the chapter on the liver (page 163).

Affirmations

- My gallbladder efficiently performs its function, so assisting and supporting the process of digestion.
- I am able to use my powers of judgement to take clear and decisive action in my life.
- I have the courage to let any repressed emotions now release in a positive and constructive manner.

See also the Liver chapter, page 178, for affirmations that may be used in conjunction with these.

Meditation for the Wood Element

Before beginning this meditation, familiarize yourself with the diagrams of the relevant meridians (i.e., for the gallbladder and liver). Remember that *qi* is pronounced 'chee', and that all meridians are bilateral (running along both sides of the body); for the purposes of this meditation the meridian points on only one side of the body are focused on. If possible, tape this meditation, reading it out clearly and slowly in a soft tone of voice.

Find a peaceful place to relax and unwind. Close your eyes. Focus your attention on your breathing and, as you begin to notice it deepening, gently let any thoughts that come into your mind float by like clouds in the sky. For a few minutes, practise the breathing exercise recommended in the lungs chapter (*page 189*).

Wood Meditation

Imagine yourself nestling between two roots of a magnificent beech tree in a beautiful woodland glade where golden shafts of light filter through the lime-green leaves. The sunlight catches the rich olive-green of new moss on the tree trunk, there is an iridescent green light and an air of stillness and peace. Notice the new growth of the leaf buds bursting open on slender young saplings which gently sway in the breeze. The atmosphere is charged with the energy and expectancy of new life, so inspiring feelings of hope, new beginnings and a fresh start. Feel the vibrant green colour which surrounds you, embracing and soothing your soul. Peace and tranquillity now flow easily through your mind, body and spirit.

Now focus your energy on your big toe, where the Liver meridian begins. Visualize the green energy flowing upwards along this meridian all the way to the right side of your ribcage where your liver and gallbladder absorb this colour. Feel it strengthening and supporting these vital organs, enabling them to perform their functions more efficiently. The meridian then goes within and travels up to your eye.

Take this green energy to the outer corner of your eye, where the Gallbladder meridian begins. Send the *qi* across your head and down the back of your neck into your shoulders and feel it releasing any tension in your muscles. See it flowing along the Gallbladder meridian running down the side of your body to the fourth toe, where the meridian ends.

Feel the surge of this Spring energy inspiring and encouraging you to make a fresh start. In your own time, begin to move your fingers and toes, feeling yourself becoming more alive, awake and full of the joys of Spring! Bring your attention back to where you are, open your eyes and stretch your body out.

The Liver

 The liver is a wedge-shaped organ situated on the right-hand side of the body beneath the diaphragm and right lung.

Western Function

The liver weighs about 1.5 kg, it is reddish-brown in colour and has two main lobes, the right lobe being six times larger than the left. It was once believed that the extent of one's health and vitality could be determined to a large degree by the health of the liver. This vital organ carries out over 500 different functions and can even regenerate its own tissue. If 90 per cent of a person's liver were removed, the remaining 10 per cent could regenerate into a complete organ!

The liver stores large quantities of nutrient-rich blood containing valuable minerals and vitamins. All the blood from the stomach and the intestines passes through the liver, allowing for full and proper absorption of nutrients. Like the spleen, the liver is an essential reservoir of the body's blood which it can release in emergencies.

The liver absorbs and stores fats, carbohydrates and proteins from our food which are then used for energy or storage in the body as fatty deposits. The liver can assist the body if it needs more immediate energy by converting stored glycogen into glucose, a simple sugar. This is sent directly into the bloodstream, to meet the body's immediate demands and keep blood sugar levels constant. Proteins are broken down and converted into their smaller components, amino acids (the nitrogenous portion not needed for new amino acids is eliminated from the body as urea).

The liver produces bile, a greenish-yellow liquid that is stored and concentrated in the gallbladder. Bile helps with the digestion and absorption of fats and stimulates the wave-like contractions called peristalsis in the large intestine. Insufficient bile can therefore contribute to constipation and digestive problems.

One of the liver's most important roles is detoxification, as it filters over a litre of blood every minute, clearing poisons, chemicals and drugs from the body and breaking these down into less toxic compounds to be easily eliminated. If the toxic load gets too high, various functions of the liver can become impaired and this can give rise to a multitude of symptoms including allergic reactions. Some classic diseases involving the liver include cirrhosis and gout, which are often caused by excessive alcohol consumption. Bruising is a sign that the liver is weak and unable to produce enough clotting factor (prothrombin). Nausea, vomiting and biliousness are other symptoms of a damaged liver, which can in turn lead to migraine. Haemorrhoids are linked with the liver: by treating this organ as well as ensuring that the bowels move regularly, haemorrhoids will often be a thing of the past.

Traditional Chinese Interpretation

Element:	Wood
Partner organ:	Gallbladder
Climate:	Wind
Season:	Spring
Colour:	Green
Time of day:	1–3 a.m.
Body tissue:	Tendons/ligaments
Voice sound:	Shouting
Sense organ:	Eyes
Reflector:	Nails
Taste:	Sour
Emotion:	Anger

SYMPTOMS OF IMBALANCE

Emotional
Anger • Irritability • Emotional repression • Depression • Inability to plan or organize • Over-fastidious planning • Impatience • Frustration • Moodiness • Rigid attitude • Negative outlook • Aggression, shouting • Nervous tension

Physical
Nausea, vomiting • Nauseous headaches, migraines • Abdominal distension, bloating • PMS, breast tenderness • Irregular, painful periods • Blurred, weak vision • Spots in front of eyes • Stiff neck, shoulders, body, muscles • Haemorrhoids • Bruising • Indigestion • Flatulence, constipation • Weak nails • Aversion to wind

---

In Chinese medicine the liver is one of the most important organs. Its key functions are seen as storing blood and ensuring the smooth flow of energy around the mind and body. When the body is at rest, the liver stores the blood and regulates the amount of blood in circulation; an inability to store and release blood contributes to stagnation of *qi* in the body. When there is a disruption of this flow of energy, many symptoms can manifest which can increase levels of both physical and mental tension within the body.

Gynaecological problems such as PMS and menstrual difficulties are linked with the liver: the meridian encircles the genital region of the body and breast tenderness can also occur if there is congestion in the liver meridian, as its pathway runs through the breasts. Lumps in the breasts and groin area can arise when there is liver stagnation. Excessive muscular tension, especially around the shoulders and neck area, is another common symptom of liver problems.

The liver can become swollen or expanded if the diet contains too many saturated fats or too much alcohol. As the organ swells, it pushes against the muscles and vertebrae, which can cause the spine to go out of alignment. Due to the relationship that the spinal nerves have to the organs, a possible cause of backache can be an imbalance in the internal organs, especially the liver, gallbladder, heart, spleen or kidneys. Backache indicating a liver imbalance is likely to be felt in the middle part of the back.

SELF-HELP FOR KEEPING YOUR LIVER HEALTHY

Chinese Nutrition

Foods for the Wood Element

Grain: wheat	Fruit: peach
Meat: chicken	Vegetable: leek

Dietary Tips

1. In early Spring (the season associated with the Wood element), eat warm foods such as stir-fries, adding more and more green vegetables that grow at this time, such as spring greens, mustard greens, romaine lettuce, radish leaves, watercress, spinach and sorrel. Include small salads in the diet again.

2. Unadulterated, unrefined, natural foods help to keep the liver healthy and efficient. A diet composed of whole grains, fresh vegetables, beans, sea vegetables (nori, wakame and kombu) and fish (the diet humans are thought to have evolved on) provides optimum nutrition without any chemical toxins or excessive fats.
3. Sesame seeds can be sprinkled over dishes and are superb for the liver as they contain protein (with eight of the important amino acids), B vitamins and vitamin E.
4. Chicory reduces heat in the liver and benefits the gallbladder. It is particularly helpful for jaundice-type hepatitis.
5. Strawberries tone the liver and kidneys, and are good for combating excessive urination and dizziness.
6. Rabbit liver is good for dizziness too and sharpens the vision.
7. Other beneficial foods for liver function are globe artichokes, asparagus, berries, buckwheat, cabbage, carrots, celery, dandelion, fennel, garlic, onion, leek, lemon, millet, oily fish, olives, parsley, parsnips, onion, brown rice, sesame oil, sunflower seeds and turmeric.
8. Wholefoods such as quinoa and amaranth are particularly beneficial for the liver.
9. A very powerful yet simple and cheap remedy to help with liver stagnation is a drink made from 240 ml hot water and 1 tablespoon of apple vinegar. One contraindication, however, is if there are a lot of heat signs within the body. A better choice would be fresh lemon juice which is a little 'cooler' energet-ically than vinegar.

Foods which are *not recommended* include alcohol, saturated fats (cheeses, cream, eggs and fat from meat), chocolate, coffee, oranges, pears, peanuts and nuts in general, sulphured dried fruits, chemical additives and refined convenience foods.

Blood-building foods
When there is a deficiency of blood in the body this can cause an imbalance in the liver as well as the brain, other vital organs, muscles and every part of us, as blood nourishes them all. The quality of blood can be improved through our diet.

- Foods rich in chlorophyll (the green substance found in leafy green vegetables), blue-green algae and spirulina, especially when combined with grains, have excellent blood-building properties.
- Beetroot is another excellent food for blood.
- Other foods which strengthen the blood are apricots, kidney beans, aduki and mung beans, dark grapes, blackstrap molasses, blackberries, nettles, parsley, watercress, eggs, figs and fish such as sardines.
- Flesh foods are well-known blood-builders; traditional Chinese medicine has it that if a particular organ is weak, you should eat more of it (for example, eating liver if your liver needs building, kidney to boost kidney energy). If you decide to follow this principle, remember that it is essential with offal, and preferably other meats too, to buy organic.

Helpful herbs and spices
- A herbal formula such as Triphala (made by Planetary formulas and available both in the UK and US) should be taken every night to ensure that toxins are removed from your system as quickly as possible.
- Parsley and dandelion are especially useful herbs for the liver and can be included in your diet, providing you can be certain that the dandelion leaves you are eating are free from pesticides. Herbalists know of their inherent value and recommend these herbs to purify the liver and 'spring clean' the blood.
- Silymarin or milk thistle has a particular affinity for the liver and can greatly assist in cleansing and supporting it.
- Herbs such as cardamom, cumin, turmeric, ginger and black pepper, as well as the condiment horseradish, can help when there is liver stagnation. Excessively hot foods (such as chilli peppers) can, however, aggravate it.
- Other beneficial culinary herbs include bay leaf, basil, rosemary and mint.
- Chamomile herbal tea (especially if brewed using the chamomile flowers themselves) is excellent for supporting liver cleansing. Peppermint tea can help to ease digestion.
- Licorice root has a real affinity with the liver and is able to

harmonize and balance liver *qi*. The root can be purchased in health food stores and chewed upon, or you can get teas with licorice in.

- Dang gui root is another liver-friendly herb which is excellent for women.
- Taking essential fatty acids in the diet is highly supportive to the liver; they are best ingested on an empty stomach first thing in the morning to help flush the liver, or taken at night before bed, as the Wood element is in power between 11 p.m. and 3 a.m.
- A useful vitamin supplement is an antioxidant formula containing selenium, vitamins C and E and beta carotene, all of which help to prevent free radical damage in the liver.
- Blue-green algae is an excellent nutrient to take to support the liver, as it not only encourages liver rejuvenation but detoxifies. Its colour is traditionally thought to reduce heat in the liver.
- Kelp is a useful supplement to take if there is liver stagnation. Alternatively, include more seaweed in your diet (*see page 167*).

Cleansing the Liver

Cleansing the liver has always been a priority in naturopathic medicine over the centuries. It is particularly beneficial for those who are sluggish, over-reactive to alcohol, intolerant to certain foods and have greeny/brown or hazel eyes (according to iridology, the practice of studying the iris of the eye to make a health diagnosis, these eye-colour types are more prone to liver and digestive disturbances). When you can no longer stand the sight or smell of fried, fatty foods, this is indeed a sign that the liver is somehow out of order. Another sign on a food front is a sudden intolerance for fruit, especially oranges, as this demonstrates that the liver has lost its ability to digest fruit acids.

Prior to working on the liver, it is highly advisable to do some work on your large intestine so that any matter that needs to be cleared in the large intestine is done so before fresh toxins are released from the liver. Liver detoxification should be undertaken gradually, as alcohol, medicines and toxins can build up over many years. The liver does not send out distress signals until a symptom or disorder has made considerable progress, so it is important to take preventative steps to support this vital organ.

'Harper's Liver Flush'
First thing every morning, drink a large fresh glass of carrot juice made with organic carrots mixed with a large tablespoon of cold-pressed oil (either olive or a mixture of oils rich in essential fatty acids) and the juice of two lemons. Blue-green algae (in capsulated form – 2–4 capsules at a time) is excellent for the liver and high in natural vitamins and minerals. Juices made with a mixture of beetroot, carrots, lemon and apple are also very beneficial. This regime should be followed for at least two weeks, preferably in the Spring or early Summer.

Exercise

We need to nurture the body and prepare it for Spring as the energy begins to rise in the body after lying dormant during the Winter months. Getting involved in gentle exercise and building your programme up over the Spring is an excellent idea; a heavy exercise regime is not recommended in the early stages of Spring. The body needs time to adapt to the new season and to allow its energy to rise up gradually from within.

Some aerobic exercise and gentle stretching to increase the oxygen intake into the muscles will be supportive when liver energy is blocked. If there is extreme stagnation and inner anger, it might be worth trying kick-boxing or investing in a punch bag to get those frustrations out of your body. Balance is the key here, as too much exercise and physical exertion is not good for any of the organs.

As a liver imbalance can generate stiffness in the body, stretching can soften the muscles and relieve built-up pressure. And just as liver congestion can cause the body to become inflexible and rigid, so stretching and softening your muscles will have a beneficial effect on your liver.

A specific exercise which stretches the liver and gallbladder meridian is described on page 153.

Touch Therapies

Reflexology

The liver reflex point is situated on the right foot. Gently massage the reflex using talc as a medium and finish by massaging your feet with a base oil (olive, sunflower, apricot, almond, etc.) to which has been added a few drops of your chosen essential oil. One or two suitable flower remedies (*see page 177*) can also be included in this mixture. For the best results, massage this into the acupressure point known as Liver 3 (*see below*) as well as the reflex point on the feet. Breathe deeply, visualizing the colour green and saying the liver sound 'SHHHHHH'. Shut out all distractions, retaining your mental tranquillity. This massage and relaxation programme will provide one of the best protective remedies for the liver. (*See page 30 for massage techniques.*)

Reflexology point for the liver (shaded)

Acupressure

The liver meridian starts on the top surface of the big toe and runs up the foot, along the inside leg, around the genitals and through the liver and gallbladder. The internal pathway of the liver meridian travels from here, up the throat until it reaches the eye (this part is not shown on the diagram).

The liver meridian

This is considered the most important point on the liver meridian. It is located in the hollow area at the top of the foot between the first and second toes, about 2.5 cm away from the webbed part. Working this point calms the nervous system, reduces irritability, strengthens the immune system and liver, prevents/relieves headaches, eases food cravings (reduces allergic sensitivity), overcomes the effects of too much exercise, stress, strains or toxins in the body and increases circulation in the legs. Using your thumb, gently rub the point, moving forwards and backwards over the area for approximately 1 to 2 minutes.

Liver 3 acupressure point (under the right thumb)

This point, right on the crown of the head, is called 'the point of a thousand meetings'; it is valuable for helping to raise and disperse liver *qi*.

Governor Vessel 20 acupressure point (draw an imaginary line from the top of the ear to the crown)

Essential Oils

Bergamot: harmonizes the liver *qi*, thus allowing an even flow of energy around the body. Regulates and calms the nervous system (nervous tension often being created by stagnation of *qi* in the liver). Helps to release pent-up feelings often experienced prior to a period, PMS being a classic example of stagnant liver energy. *Strength factor: Medium*

Bitter orange: unblocks stagnant *qi* when it builds in the liver, stomach and intestines, thereby easing emotional tension, difficulty sleeping/insomnia and nauseous headaches or migraines. Ideal for digestive symptoms such as abdominal distension, flatulence, indigestion, nausea, vomiting and constipation. Stimulates the liver and the gallbladder, encouraging the flow of bile and thus supporting the body with the breakdown of fats. Can be useful for workaholic types who are intolerant of mistakes. Works well with the Bach Flower Remedy Rock Water (*see page 177*). Tangerine also regulates *qi* and helps alleviate nausea. *Strength factor: Medium*

Chamomile: eases emotional tension, frustration and depression. If the *qi* is very stuck, it can affect the flow of blood, leading to a condition known as 'blood stagnation' in Chinese medicine. This can create menstrual disorders and pain, but Chamomile's superb analgesic properties can help to reduce this pain. *Strength factor: Strong*

Grapefruit: cools an over-heated and abused liver. Detoxifies and cleanses the body; boosts a sluggish lymphatic system. Has a wonderful fruity, uplifting smell that can ease frustration and tension. For those with eating disorders or those who raid the refrigerator when under pressure, this oil erases the guilt, self-blame, remorse and depression that follows a 'binge'. Heals that vulnerable inner part of ourselves that was crying out for help in the first place. *Strength factor: Medium*

Lavender: clears anger from the liver and cleanses and soothes the spirit of anger and exhaustion. Has nerve-relaxant properties, making it ideal for releasing liver stagnation, which upsets the flow of body energy and blood and gives rise to frustration, mood swings, anger, abdominal distension, headaches and menstrual disorders. Just as it can soothe the discomfort of sunburn, lavender can also disperse some of the latent heat that can build up in the liver and generate further stagnation, as well as diffuse overheated emotions. *Strength factor: Weak*

Neroli: calms the mind, relaxes the nervous system, gently lifts the spirit. Particularly comforting to 'sensitive souls' who have the tendency to over-work and drive themselves too hard, falling prey to mental and emotional exhaustion. Comforts and strengthens the mind, body and spirit, bringing them back to a point of balance and harmony. *Strength factor: Medium*

Emotions

Anger is the emotion connected to the liver – not surprisingly, the sound associated with the liver is shouting. One of the biochemical jobs of the liver is to absorb nutrients from the blood and store them. Emotionally, it is thought to play a similar role, as it is believed to 'absorb anger', preventing us from becoming depressed and overwrought. However, when there is obstruction of feelings and chronic bottled-up frustration, this may well result in anger alternating with depression. A depression of a liver nature invariably follows periods of long-term stress and pressure which ultimately take their toll on the individual.

Addictions are closely related to the liver, be they related to alcohol, drugs or food. The emotional tension that gives rise to addictions is felt in the liver. As the liver is a powerful detoxifying plant, it becomes a dumping ground for those poisonous aspects of our being which we feel we cannot express: hatred, envy, rage, jealousy and self-disgust. If these emotions accumulate in the liver, they will weaken it and impair its function. If negative feelings and thoughts build up, this can have a detrimental affect on the immune system and the body's ability to cope with infections. The energy generated from particular repressed emotions accumulates in the form of tension and bunched muscles in our shoulders, neck and back. When the emotion is anger, the specific sentiment associated with the liver and gallbladder, backache can occur in the middle part of the back.

Coming to terms with anger and feeling OK about releasing this is an important part of getting better. Sometimes it may not be advisable to let your frustrations out in a public way. In these cases, find somewhere quiet and private, then re-enact the scenario that led to your frustration and anger. Visualize the person or situation and say exactly what you would have liked to have said earlier on, no holds barred! Alternatively, writing your feelings down on paper in the form of a letter could be helpful. You are not actually going to send it to the person concerned, so give full vent to your anger. If your emotions are severely repressed and you cannot even get in touch with your anger (another sign of an imbalance of the liver), it may be worth seeing a fully trained counsellor who can help you to get in touch with these feelings and learn to express them.

When liver *qi* starts to stagnate due to frustrations at home, work or school, an excellent way of handling them is to go to a quiet space and physically get the anger out by punching the air, a pillow or the bed, or stamping your feet and punching your fists out at the same time. Making the sound 'HO HO HO HO HO' (a technique used by certain Native American tribes; *see page 158*), in a very definite and powerful voice (not the jolly 'ho ho ho' that Santa Claus makes!), also works wonders.

The liver is known as the body's planner or internal filofax, together with its partner organ the gallbladder, which is responsible for decision-making. If there is any stagnation in the liver, then both indecisive and disorganized behaviour will be apparent. So any problems relating to either poor planning and time management, or conversely being a fanatical filofax freak and meticulously planning everything to the last detail, can point to a liver imbalance.

On a more spiritual level, the liver is where the *Hun* or spiritual soul lives. The *Hun* hates alcohol, poisons and emotions such as anger; when these are present the *Hun* is said to flee from the body, which can be disastrous! However, good deeds and acts of compassion will encourage it to return! The 'Hun' or soul thrives on having a sense of purpose and vision; without these it becomes discontented and despairing, stagnation of liver *qi* contributing to this loss of aspiration and motivation. At this level, certain oils and flower remedies can be extremely beneficial in bringing harmony back to mind, body and spirit (*see page 174 and below*).

Flower Remedies

Impatiens: for mood swings, impatience, anger, inner tension, a 'blowing hot and cold' disposition, over-reactions and general irritability. Eases these 'pressure cooker' feelings and generates empathy, compassion, gentleness and understanding for others.

Rock Water: for perfectionist individuals who constantly drive and strive and thus become over-tense and irritable. These types can be so strict and inflexible they deny themselves any pleasures, thus creating even more liver *qi* stagnation. This is a good remedy to add to your bath water (about 6 drops, possibly along with Bitter orange essential oil, which complements Rock Water well).

Vervain: For workaholic type personalities prone to overexertion who set up stress patterns in the body typical of liver symptoms (including headaches, physical tension, muscle congestion, migraines and eyestrain). Allows us to become more tolerant of situations, to let go and go with the flow. Channels our natural enthusiasms and leads to an altogether more calm, relaxed life.

You may also find some appropriate flower remedies for supporting the Wood element in the chapter on the gallbladder (page 126).

Affirmations

- I respect and entrust my liver to perform its many varied and complex functions.
- I feel calm, confident and able to organize and plan my life.
- I am flexible and yielding, my body moves with grace and ease.
- The life force (or *qi*) moves freely throughout my mind and body, dispersing any congestion.
- I fill my liver with a healing green light which calms my spirit, dissolves tension and fills me with a sense of peace and wellbeing.

See also the Gallbladder chapter, page 159, for affirmations that may be used in conjunction with these.

Meditation for the Wood Element
See Gallbladder chapter, page 160.

The Metal Element

Partner Organs: The lungs and large intestine are the partner organs for the Metal element. The lungs expel carbon dioxide, and the large intestine eliminates solid residue. If this waste is not eliminated frequently it can have an effect on the skin. The skin is known in TCM as 'the third lung'; it is part of the Metal element and can reflect sluggish bowels (toxins that remain in the colon for too long will be discharged through the skin). The bowel is one of the most important routes of elimination for self-cleansing, and works together with the kidneys, bladder, lungs and skin to help eliminate waste efficiently from the body. It contains friendly bacteria which can synthesize B vitamins and help to keep the level of harmful, pathogenic bacteria to a minimum.

Climate: Dryness: a passion for dry weather or, conversely, a hatred of it point to a Metal element imbalance. In nature, Autumn reflects dryness, as seen in the leaves when they lose their moisture, shrivel up and 'let go' of the branches they have hung on to since Springtime.

Season: Autumn, the time to reflect on the past year and to prepare for withdrawing as the Winter months close in. It is a time to protect the back of the neck from the winds, which begin to get cooler, otherwise you will be more susceptible to minor illnesses after the hot Summer months.

Colour: White. Someone obsessed with wearing white or who strongly dislikes the colour can be demonstrating an imbalance in the Metal element. A white hue coming off the face is also indicative of lung problems according to TCM, just as a very white or pale skin in Western medicine is considered a sign that the lungs are too tight or there is local congestion, constricting the circulation.

Time of Day: 3–5 a.m. (lungs): if there are problems with this organ you may wake up between these times and even experience breathing difficulties. This shows that there are unresolved issues around the emotion of grief, which corresponds to the Metal element. Extreme grief is injurious to the lungs, and a person who is going through a period of grieving will often have bowel problems. The time of day for the large intestine is 5–7 a.m.; according to TCM this is the best time of day to have your first bowel movement. If there are any imbalances in the bowel, getting up between these times will encourage the body to rid itself efficiently of toxins held in the bowel.

Body Tissue: The skin is seen as the third lung and breathes just as surely and necessarily as the lungs themselves. The link between lung problems and the skin is quite well documented in Western medicine; it is common for children who have been given suppressive skin treatments for eczema to go on to develop asthma. It is known that many skin problems such as psoriasis, eczema, rough, dry skin and rashes reflect an imbalance in the body that relates directly to the lungs. The correlation of the skin with the lungs and respiratory function is an important diagnostic tool in Chinese medicine. Elimination is also associated with the skin, since the skin is involved in the process of ridding the body of wastes. In Japan there is also an ancient belief that the skin reflects the condition of the internal organs: if the latter are fatigued in any way, it will reflect on our skin.

Voice Sound: The sound of the Metal element is a weeping tone of voice, which does not always coincide with actual tears. There is often a sense of sadness and loss, grief being the emotion of the Metal element. The voice will invariably be very soft, too, almost angelic or ethereal.

Sense Organ: We usually breathe through the nose. In TCM, the lungs are never separated from the nose, which is the sense organ of the Metal element. Problems which affect the nose have a direct bearing on the lungs; equally, lung problems are often accompanied by disturbances in the nasal fluids. The secretion for this element is mucus, from any of the mucus membranes in the body. A deficiency of mucus can show that the body is overheated, causing dryness on the surface of the skin. Alternatively, an excessive amount of mucus indicates an imbalance in the lungs. Therefore, dryness in the throat or nose, coughing, difficulty breathing, aching in the lungs, rasping, nasal drip and sinus blockages can all be related to the Metal element. Often your sense of smell is affected when the energy in the Metal element is not properly balanced.

Reflector: Body hair is the physical manifestation of the Metal element. Excessive body hair or the loss of body hair points to an imbalance. The hair on our head, however, is ruled by the kidneys.

Symptoms of Imbalance: Oedema, wet skin, excessive mucus and abnormal perspiration patterns are connected with the lungs, as the lungs, along with the Water element, play an important role in the regulation of body fluids. Conversely, deficiencies of moisture can cause severe dryness in the body, signs of which may be lack of secretions, emaciation, anaemia, poor appetite and a white, ethereal appearance. The skin will be tight and therefore perspiration sparse. The large intestine has the ability, on a higher level, to generate movement forwards in our lives, encouraging evolution and change. Constriction and cynical behaviour patterns emerge if the energy of the large intestine is poor. In TCM, nose bleeds, sore throat, neck swelling, thirst and a dry mouth, toothache and pain along the relevant meridian are all symptoms of an imbalance in the large intestine. When there are intestinal disorders, including chronic constipation, the blood can become congested in the colon.

The Lungs

 The lungs are cone-shaped organs located inside the rib cage and separated from the abdominal organs by a sheet of muscle called the diaphragm.

Western Function

The main function of the lungs is to supply the body with oxygen, which is transported through the circulatory system in the blood. The 'used' air, which is composed of toxins and carbon dioxide, is released by the lungs when we exhale.

Good lung ventilation is assured by clean air and healthy lung tissue. Sadly, with our environmental conditions worsening year by year, the functioning of our lungs is often impaired. Every part of our body, from our organs to our blood and cells, can be poisoned by what is absorbed from the external environment. Our internal environment can also have a great impact on our lungs. Emotional stresses can result in constriction of the lungs, thus preventing an efficient changeover of nutrients in the blood.

Weakness in the lungs manifest in susceptibility to asthma, emphysema, bronchitis and infections of the throat, sinuses and chest. Air pollution and high stress levels can weaken the immune system and lungs and contribute to allergic reactions such as hayfever and asthma. Having very white or pale skin can indicate a deficiency of haemoglobin (the protein that carries oxygen and iron) in the blood and possibly lung weakness. Smoking injures the lungs and creates heat and dryness; excessive consumption of fat also weakens the lungs as too much cholesterol and fat in the bloodstream reduce the oxygen-carrying capacity of the blood. The dangers of smoking are well documented, but one interesting fact that is not so widely known is that smokers mix tiny amounts of nicotine into their saliva. This then has an impact on digestion as it inhibits the production of gastric juices in the stomach.

Traditional Chinese Interpretation

Element:	Metal
Partner organ:	Large intestine
Climate:	Dryness
Season:	Autumn
Colour:	White
Time of day:	3–5 a.m.
Body tissue:	Skin
Voice sound:	Weeping
Sense organ:	Nose
Reflector:	Body Hair
Taste:	Spicy
Emotion:	Grief

SYMPTOMS OF IMBALANCE

Emotional
Grief • Being unable to let go • Apathy, boredom • Lack of inspiration • Melancholy • Pessimism • Remote, distant behaviour

---

In traditional Chinese medicine it is believed that the lungs extract
clean *qi* from the inhaled air and combine this with food *qi* from
the spleen. The lungs spread *qi* all over the body to nourish the
tissues and promote all physiological processes. The lungs govern
the breath and are responsible for the production of 'defensive *qi*'.
This *qi* is said to protect us from damaging external climatic factors
such as wind, cold and damp, to which the lungs are quite
vulnerable. The lungs disperse this 'defensive *qi*' to fluids found in
the spaces between the skin and muscles throughout the body. This
function ensures defensive *qi* is equally distributed under the skin
and can perform its role in warming the skin and muscles, so
protecting the body. If the lung energy is weak, our resistance will
be lowered and we will be more prone to infections.

The respiratory function affects all the rhythms of the
body/mind, including blood flow. Breathing, along with food, is
one of the main ways to replenish the body and its energy levels.
However, because it is so simple and basic to life, breathing often
can be overlooked until a specific problem arises such as asthma
or shortness of breath.

The highest function of the lungs, according to the Chinese, is
that they act as the Receiver of Energy, taking energy from the
outside into ourselves, on every level. We breathe emotionally as
well as physically – the expressions *breathless with excitement*
and *breathtaking* give us a hint of this. The larynx is part of the
respiratory system, so the lung meridian controls the voice.
When your tone of voice is quiet, this can indicate that the state
of *qi* within the body is quite deficient.

SELF-HELP FOR KEEPING YOUR LUNGS HEALTHY

Nutrition

Foods for the Metal Element

Grain: rice	Fruit: chestnut
Meat: horse*	Vegetable: onions

If an element is out of balance, the right foods help restore it. A combination of foods for all the elements is a healthy, balanced diet.

Dietary Tips

1. The flavour associated with the Metal element is pungent and spicy, referring to curries, spices and peppery foods. Excess pungent foods make the muscles knotty and the finger and toe nails weak, according to ancient Chinese texts. The pungency goes directly to the respiratory tract, so it is important to moderate your intake of these foods. However, other organs can benefit from this flavour: if, for example, the kidneys suffer from dryness, pungent foods will moisten them.
2. Common foods in Chinese medicine to enhance lung function are carrots, button mushrooms, crab apples, olives, pears, radishes, tangerines, walnuts, water chestnuts and wine.
3. Peaches and green onions are known to stop perspiration.
4. Other supportive foods are watercress, mustard and cress, turnips, Chinese cabbage and celery. Apples, apricots, egg whites, mandarins, strawberries and peanuts all help to lubricate the lungs.
5. Dairy products (especially taken cold) and orange juice should be avoided if there is any sign of mucus in the body, as they can increase mucus production.

* While horse meat is recommended for this element, I do not condone its consumption.

Helpful herbs and spices

- Garlic has a direct affinity with the lungs: if you rub your feet with a clove of garlic, in 15 minutes your breath will smell of garlic! It can also help to reduce the amount of mucus produced by the body.
- Ginger is used for any condition where the body is not coping effectively with balancing its moisture levels; it can help to dry up excess mucus.
- There is a remedy called Trikatu (made with ginger root and black pepper) which can dry up excessive amounts of mucus in the body (available from *Planetary Formulas*).
- 'Yogi tea', which contains cloves, cinnamon, cardamom, ginger and black pepper, is very useful if you are coming down with a cold.
- Basil and peppermint enhance lung function.
- Cinnamon induces perspiration, as does coriander, fresh ginger, rosemary and marjoram.
- Ginseng helps to lubricate the lungs.

Exercise

Vigorous cardiovascular exercise obviously has a beneficial effect on the lungs as breathing becomes more frequent and deeper. Too much lying down can damage the lung and large intestine meridians, affecting both elimination and respiration. To remedy this, work on acupressure point Large Intestine 4, located in the muscle between the thumb and first finger, and on Large Intestine 11, found at the elbow crease on the outer part of the arm (*see Figure, page 211*).

The stretch for the lung and large intestine meridians involves clasping your hands behind your back and bending forward gently, keeping your knees unlocked. Lift your arms as high as possible behind you. Hold and breathe deeply. Repeat three times then relax; follow with some deep breathing exercises. Remember that it may take weeks or months to achieve this. Work at your own pace and ensure that you have warmed the muscles in your body for 10 minutes prior to stretching. If possible, join a local yoga class where you can be guided and personally instructed.

The lung/large intestine stretch

Breathing Exercises

Breathing exercises are an essential part of any self-healing programme. The rise and the fall of the lungs and diaphragm will directly affect the internal organs positively, as the movement massages them internally. Practising this on a daily basis, along with following the other guidelines recommended in this book, will keep the internal organs in top form.

Deep breathing gives us the breath of life and puts us in touch with ourselves. It is believed to be the interface between body and mind. Learning how to breathe deeply and fully can help us to experience a new awakening of energy and a greater enthusiasm for life. Conversely, shallow breathing or breathing difficulties can cause the body to become sluggish and toxic, hampering the healing process. It is essential that the organs, tissues and cells all receive an adequate supply of oxygen to allow them to carry out their duties efficiently.

Lying or sitting in a comfortable position, place one hand on your lower abdomen and one on your chest. Take a slow, deep breath, allowing the air to flow down to your abdomen. Feel your lower hand rise as the air fills this area. At the same time, notice whether there is much movement of the hand that is on your chest. The ultimate aim is that the hand on your abdomen should rise and fall with your breathing, while the hand on your chest remains relatively still. Exhale slowly, allowing your abdomen and lungs to deflate properly. Again, focus on your lower hand rising as you inhale fresh, clean air. Hold the breath for a few seconds and, on exhaling, allow your abdomen to collapse, ensuring that all the stale air that you have been storing in your body is released. Do this three times and then relax into a natural pattern of breathing.

If there is grieving or sadness, back pain will be felt between the shoulder blades. Massaging the sternum can also help, using small circular movements, noting any sensitive spots and gently working on them (*see Heart chapter, page 89*).

Touch Therapies

Reflexology

The ball of the foot is the area that connects to the lungs; as we have both a right and a left lung, the points are found on both feet. Holding your left foot, massage the ball of the foot, noting any sore areas or gritty parts. These 'crystals' are a build-up of uric acid that can quite easily break down. However, don't endeavour to get rid of them all in one or two sessions. Try and massage your foot every day or every other day, just for a couple of minutes. (*See page 30 for massage techniques.*)

Reflexology points for the lungs (shaded)

When doing any of the above exercises, always make the lung sound 'SSSSSSS' as you exhale, slowly controlling your breath and visualizing a white, healing light flowing in during inhalation. See it entering your lungs and permeating the oxygen molecules so that this white light is carried all around the body, thus promoting healing on a very deep level.

Acupressure

The meridian for the lungs has an internal branch which begins near the stomach and goes upwards through the upper body cavity, surfacing below the clavicle (Lung 1). It then descends the lateral side of the left arm and finishes on the outside of the thumb nail.

lung 1

The lung meridian

Acupressure has been found to be extremely beneficial for most lung imbalances. A study of asthma patients in the US revealed that their lung capacity increased after a 20-minute acupressure session.

LUNG 1

This point is found on the outer part of the chest, about 2.5–5 cm beneath the collarbone. It is one of the main points to help release tension caused by emotional stress. Holding it relieves difficult breathing and asthma symptoms, and releases suppressed grief.

LUNG 7

This point greatly strengthens the lungs and entire respiratory system. It is located 2.5 cm from the wrist crease on the inside of the forearm, in line with the thumb. It is a good preventative point for breathing difficulties and congestion, and also helps to relieve coughs and colds, especially in the early stages. It can help to revitalize and lift the spirits, as it helps to move and circulate lung *qi*. It is also a useful point for easing a runny nose and correcting a loss of the sense of smell.

Essential Oils

Clary Sage: strengthens lung energy and soothes a constricted chest. Restores our inner reserves when they are weak and vulnerable. Contains the plant hormones known as phyto-oestrogens, so use with care. *Strength factor: Strong*

Cypress: strengthens and supports the Bodily Soul and heavenly *qi*. Relaxes breathing and encourages us to flow on an emotional level, taking in the new and releasing the old. Helps in times of change and upheaval. *Strength factor: Medium*

Eucalyptus: a classic respiratory oil which has a very strong connection to the lung area. Anticatarrhal, antibacterial and anti-viral; unmatched for its powerful action on lung infections, sinusitis and even the common cold. Clears mucus and decongests both the lungs and whole body,

Lung 7 acupressure point

supporting and enhancing immune system functioning. Lifts the spirits, dispersing any negative feelings of suffocation, melancholy and grief. Brings a sense of release, so allowing life to move forward once again. *Strength factor: Strong*

Frankincense: strengthens the defensive *qi* and so greatly supports and protects the immune system. Calming, helping to deepen the breath and slow down respiration. Ideal for asthma, as it can help to relieve tightness in the chest, and for conditions such as bronchitis. Possesses expectorant and anti-catarrhal properties. *Strength factor: Strong*

Pine: like Eucalyptus, another lung oil which is excellent in fighting off colds and lung infections. If lung function is weak, you are more vulnerable to these infections; Pine, being a herb of protection, would be useful in a blend, or added to your bath. *Strength factor: Medium*

Tea Tree: possesses supreme antifungal and antiviral properties together with being a powerful natural antibiotic. Strengthens weak lung *qi*, thus easing symptoms such as shallow breathing, chronic weakness, mental fatigue and general immune disorders. Increases our resistance to disease so is a perfect choice for vulnerable, weak, susceptible individuals who are prone to catching common infections. Can help to boost morale after a debilitating illness. *Strength factor: Strong*

Thyme: an extremely 'hot' anti-infectious oil that has a very invigorating effect on both the physical and mental plane. Uplifts, tones and strengthens weak lung energy; can help to ease conditions such as chronic fatigue syndrome, white or clear catarrh and coughs, and opens the chest thus helping improve shallow breathing. Lifts us out of melancholy and grief by enhancing the heavenly *qi*. *Strength factor: Strong*

It is always best to seek advice from a trained aromatherapist or herbalist who can assess your individual needs. For example, with a condition such as asthma, the choice of oils could depend on whether the asthma was emotionally based or caused by an allergy or infection.

Other oils of benefit include Rose, Lavender, Neroli, Chamomile and Bergamot (for their anti-spasmodic, anti-inflammatory and anti-depressant properties), along with Sandalwood, Marjoram, Myrrh and Benzoin.

Emotions

Traditional Chinese medicine associates prolonged sorrow and grief with the lungs. Grief is a natural, human emotion like all the emotions we experience, but someone who is constantly overwhelmed by sorrow is considered to be suffering an imbalance afflicting the organs of the Metal element.

The lungs are very much involved with the process of 'letting go'. After all, if the lungs did not 'let go' of the carbon dioxide and other toxins that are expelled during expiration, then we *would* be in trouble! The letting go of emotions, grief and sadness has just as much relevance: if these emotions are held inside over time, then we put ourselves at risk of developing physical ailments.

The lungs receive what is termed as 'heavenly *qi*', thought to provide inspiration and a sense of meaning in life. If the energy flow is poor, apathy, boredom and a lack of inspiration and meaning in life may be the result. The Bodily Soul, or *P'o* as it is called by the Chinese, is believed to live in the lungs and is easily affected by negative emotions, especially those of remorse and pessimism. If one has never truly grieved over a loss, it can develop into a Metal element depression which manifests as an inability to progress in life.

Flower Remedies

Honeysuckle: for those who just cannot seem to move on; a good remedy for grief as it helps to dissolve remorse and regrets about the past. Makes us feel more focused and aware of the present. Can also be used for childhood traumas that haunt you, and in times of bereavement where it is extremely difficult to get over the loss of a loved one.

Hornbeam: the remedy for that 'Monday morning feeling', when you feel lethargic, weary, apathetic, unmotivated and bored. Helps to encourage us to face the day with renewed vigour and a freshness of mind and body. Revitalizes and strengthens the heavenly *qi*, thus providing more meaning and inspiration in your life.

Pine: has a highly therapeutic action on the lungs. Recommended for people who blame themselves and carry guilt, feeling responsible for the actions of others. Helps to dissolve guilt and remorse and enables us to distinguish when a problem is ours and when it is someone else's.

Water Violet: for those who withdraw into their own little world for protection. They cannot let people into their space or 'receive' the richness of human experience and advice. Helps to break down the walls that surround them, allowing others to come closer and yet still retain their serenity and poise.

Wild Rose: for dullness and fatigue when the energy flow of heavenly *qi* is low and there is no sense of meaning in life. Revives the spirit and renews our sense of joy, bringing new levels of inspiration and motivation.

You may also find some appropriate flower remedies for supporting the Metal element in the chapter in the large intestine (page 213).

Affirmations

- I now expand my lungs and breathe deeply, so inhaling the sustaining breath of life.
- With every breath I take, I feel protected and uplifted by the life force.
- I now let go of any sadness and pain that I have experienced in my past.
- I am filled with inspiration and divine energy.

See also the Large Intestine chapter, page 110, for affirmations that may be used in conjunction with these.

Meditation for the Metal Element

Before beginning this meditation exercise, familiarize yourself with the diagrams of the relevant meridians (i.e. for the lungs and large intestine). Remember that *qi* is pronounced 'chee', and that all meridians are bilateral (running along both sides of the body); for the purposes of this meditation the meridian points on only one side of the body are focused on. If possible, tape this meditation, reading it out clearly and slowly in a soft tone of voice.

Find a peaceful place to relax and unwind. Close your eyes. Focus your attention on your breathing and, as you begin to notice it deepening, gently let any thoughts that come into your mind float by like clouds in the sky. For a few minutes, practise the breathing exercise recommended in the Lung chapter (*page 187*).

Metal Meditation

Imagine yourself sitting beneath the boughs of a mighty oak tree in Autumn. Notice the leaves on the different trees in the wood and see the rich variations in colour from red to russet and gold set against the early evening sky. This time of year represents the drawing in and bringing to a close the earlier seasons of growth and abundance. Just as Nature has to let go of her fruits and leaves, so you too can begin to let go of ideas and thoughts which are outmoded and no longer have relevance in your life.

Focus more closely on a branch of a tree with its leaves about to fall. As you watch, a yellow leaf falls gently to the earth. Imagine that this falling leaf represents a feeling, an event or a relationship that you need to release. Allow yourself to experience this loss and give thanks that you have been able to let it go. Continue this process of attaching emotions or events to various leaves on the branch until you feel that you have let go of the negative thoughts and feelings which are no longer necessary in your life.

Now visualize a beautiful white light entering the top of your head. Feel this healing white light as it gently cleanses your mind, and know inside that by releasing the old, you have created room for new, fresh and positive thoughts and feelings. Feel the sense of peace, clarity and calmness that this realization brings. In your own time, allow the white light to flow down into your neck and shoulders, releasing any stiffness held in this area of your body. Now concentrate and intensify the white light in your lungs. When you feel ready, visualize the *qi* flowing from the lungs towards the Lung meridian, beginning on the front of your shoulder. Send the white light down the inside of your arm until it reaches the inside of your thumb. Next, allow the *qi* to flow up your index finger, where the Large Intestine meridian begins, along the outside of your arm, over your shoulder and on to its finishing point near the outer part of your nose.

Feeling more relaxed and refreshed, with your breathing becoming deeper and steadier with every inhalation, allow the white light to flow down to your large intestine. Intensify the light and feel it cleansing your body of all the mental and physical toxins stored in your colon. Allow these to be dissolved by the white light and imagine that this then flows down your legs and out through your toes to be transmuted by the earth.

When you feel ready, begin to move your fingers and toes, feeling yourself becoming more alive and refreshed. Slowly bring your attention back to where you are, open your eyes and stretch your body out.

The Large Intestine

 The large intestine or colon is a muscular tube about 1.5 m long. It is located in the lower abdominal region and is the last section of the digestive tract.

Western Function

Its prime function is to eliminate the by-products of digestion (the faeces) and to absorb water through the walls of the colon, so helping to conserve body fluids. The first half of this tube absorbs water from waste products, the second half acts as a storage depot for the faeces before they are expelled by the anus.

The residues of digested food empty from the small intestine into the colon in a liquid form. Peristalsis (muscular wave-like contractions of the intestine) squeezes moisture from the waste at regular intervals. This is reabsorbed back into the body and the faeces move along the length of the colon, helped by these contractions. The indigestible waste material is now relatively compact and is stored until it is time to be expelled via the anus.

The large intestine is divided into three sections: the ascending colon, transverse colon and descending colon. The ascending colon extends up the right side of the abdomen to a point near the liver (known as the hepatic flexure). From here it travels across the body (thus being termed the transverse colon) to a point on the left-hand side near the spleen (the splenic flexure). Then, like the descending colon, it travels down the left-hand side of the body, turns towards the centre of the body, leads to the rectum and finally the anus. If you ever massage your colon, always follow this natural (clockwise) direction – otherwise you will be pushing the contents the wrong way!

The appendix is another part of the colon, considered to have no real significance today by the medical profession. However, the appendix has been recognized in the East for thousands of years as playing a vital role in our immune system. This is because the appendix secretes a fluid containing anti-bacterial, antifungal and antiviral substances; this fluid also helps to lubricate the waste material, thus reducing the chance of it stagnating in the colon.

The ileocaecal valve is located at the beginning of the ascending colon and separates the small and large intestines.

Traditional Chinese Interpretation

Element:	Metal
Partner organ:	Lungs
Climate:	Dryness
Season:	Autumn
Colour:	White
Time of day:	5–7 a.m.
Body tissue:	Skin
Voice sound:	Weeping
Sense organ:	Nose
Reflector:	Body Hair
Taste:	Spicy
Emotion:	Grief

The large intestine continually takes in food and 'transports, transforms and eliminates'. It has a direct impact on and complementary relationship with its partner organ, the lungs, because if there is excess *qi* in the large intestine this travels upwards to the lungs.

When the colon is out of balance, the whole body is affected. Toxic wastes build up and can eventually filter back into the system. Toxins stored in the body will make the skin more coarse and your body more likely to experience aches and pains. Symptoms such as constipation, diarrhoea, flatulence and lower abdominal pain are obvious signs to watch out for. Also, abdominal distension, bad breath, haemorrhoids and poor memory can indicate a sluggish colon. There is also a close relationship between body odour and toxins in the colon. If someone, no matter how frequently they wash, cannot control their body odour and the smell of their feet, this can illustrate that the colon is not in good shape. Flatulence arises when one or more of the digestive organs such as the stomach, liver, gallbladder, small intestine or pancreas is not secreting sufficient digestive juices, and can disappear when a proper diet is followed and intestinal function is restored.

SELF-HELP FOR HEALING YOUR LARGE INTESTINE

Chinese Nutrition

Foods for the Metal Element

Grain: rice	Fruit: chestnut
Meat: horse	Vegetable: onions

The most important foods for colon maintenance and cleansing are vegetables and fibre. Cellulose, the structural material of vegetables and fruit, is a very dense form of carbohydrate which has the ability to stimulate and enhance the function of the intestine. With all the curves and bends in the intestine, wastes can become lodged, creating pockets in the bowels (known as diverticulitis) where bacteria can flourish. We have forgotten how to feed our colons, they have been made redundant with all the fast and refined foods that are part of the nineties diet. Many medical researchers believe that cancer and other diseases of the colon can be prevented with a diet containing large amounts of vegetable fibre. Fibre is needed to speed the expulsion process in the colon; if absent from the diet, colon contents stagnate and the disease process can begin.

Foods that contain a high proportion of water are also important, as are those with either a neutral pH or an alkaline pH. This is because our body's acid-alkaline balance is often 80 per cent acid/20 per cent alkaline when it should ideally be 80 per cent alkaline/20 per cent acid! Vegetables are wonderfully alkaline foods, so include them in abundance in your diet, and especially if you suffer from problems with the large intestine. The exceptions are members of the nightshade family of vegetables – potatoes, tomatoes, aubergines, peppers, as well as tobacco – which contain a toxin called solanine to which individuals suffering from body pain and arthritis are very sensitive. Citrus fruits are also best avoided by those sensitive individuals whose digestive system cannot tolerate anything too acidic.

Unless you already consume large amounts of raw foods, start slowly and gently with any cleansing programme. Raw fruit and honey are especially 'aggressive' cleansers. Some vegetables also have a strong cleansing action, so these too are best eaten in moderation in the early stages – onions, leeks, chives, fenugreek and turnips.

For the average person, this is not always the best way to start a cleansing programme as it can swing the body into 'shock cleansing'. This is because toxins are stored in the body in the deep organs such as the liver and kidneys. When you go on to a raw cleansing diet, the toxins are brought up from these organs to the superficial systems of elimination, where the bowel, skin and lymphatic system all play crucial roles. However, if these systems have not been prepared in advance for such a cleansing, it can put considerable strain on the organs in the body and trigger a 'healing crisis'. A cleansing reaction or healing crisis occurs when toxic substances are expelled from the body tissues faster than the organs of elimination can remove them, leading to toxicity in the blood and lymph.

In Chinese medicine, raw food is seen to weaken the spleen. This can make the body more prone to being 'cold and damp' with symptoms such as water retention, slightly sticky hands, abdominal distension and loose stools. If you are really hooked on raw food, then at least create some balance by warming your body up with herbs such as ginger and cinnamon. See the chapter on the spleen (*page 69*) for other food recommendations.

The Chinese believe that eating more refined foods and fewer fibre and vegetables causes us to have less *qi*. Toxins build up inside the body and begin to poison our system by a process known as 'auto-intoxication' where the body reabsorbs toxins from the waste lying in the colon. This affects the liver and symptoms can include anything from mood changes and irritability to more chronic conditions. The blood is also affected, as the liver's filtering job is impaired, which can have a negative effect on the whole body.

Dietary Tips

1. Aduki beans, aubergines, bean curd, cauliflower, celery, Chinese cabbage, corn, cucumber, figs, honey, lettuce, onions and yellow

soya beans are some of the foods recommended by traditional Chinese medicine to support the colon.

2. Increase consumption of grains such as rice and millet. Millet is a gluten-free, alkaline grain which does not create mucus in the body. However, it can be very stodgy if not prepared correctly. Soak it overnight and rinse well, then simmer for 10 minutes, watching carefully that it doesn't get too thick. It does have a rather bland taste (that's putting it politely!) and is best added to flavoursome soups or tossed into a stir-fry with plenty of garden herbs.

3. Avoid wheat bran, as it can scratch the lining of the large intestine. Whole grain oats are a better source of fibre and are kinder on the colon. Wheat bran is also high in a substance known as phytate or phytic acid, which has the capacity to bind to minerals such as calcium and magnesium, thus preventing the body from absorbing them. The absorption of zinc and iron may also be impaired in this way.

4. Increase your vegetable intake: steam or stir-fry them with seaweed and spices such as ginger and garlic. Try vegetable soups. You can stir-fry without oil – sweat an onion in a small amount of water. Once the onion has released its juices, add spices and herbs, followed by the vegetables.

5. Avocado, sprouting seeds and pulses make excellent and highly nutritious ingredients in any meal.

6. Milk and dairy products are not viewed as particularly beneficial to the colon as they can bring on diarrhoea and vomiting in susceptible individuals and contribute towards congestion. If you are not sensitive to dairy products, the addition of live natural yoghurt (made from either cow's, goat's or sheep's milk) can replenish the amount of the valuable lactobacillus acido-philus bacteria in the colon, so helping to keep levels of putrefactive bacteria down.

7. Pomegranates can be very irritating to the colon and should be avoided. Nuts should not be eaten if you suffer from diverticulitis.

8. Cocoa, tea and coffee contain caffeine which can contribute to gastric troubles, ulcers and indigestion. The aromatic oils in coffee can cause diarrhoea; the tannin in tea induces constipation. Tea, coffee, chocolate, soft drinks and alcohol are diuretics, removing fluids and minerals from the body and causing dehydration.

9. Air pollution, smoking and central heating and travelling also contribute to dehydration. It is essential, therefore, to drink plenty of water. Remember, in the colder months, to drink warm water (never iced water).
10. Eat only moderate amounts of animal protein (meat and poultry) if you are very constipated, as it can slow down the process of peristalsis in the intestine. Make vegetables and rice the main part of your meals, with meat as a 'side dish'.
11. Soya beans are mucus-forming and intake should be limited. However, if the beans are sprouted for six days they lose their mucus properties.

Helpful herbs and spices
- Basil is helpful for constipation.
- Ginger root, black pepper, nutmeg, garlic, mustard greens and daikon radish are medicinal herbs for the Metal element.
- Psyllium husks are classically used in bowel formulae as they swell with water, forming a wallpaper-like solution, and are unsurpassed at loosening old matter and increasing the size of the bulky mass travelling though the intestine. However, it is of a 'cool' nature according to food energetics; reputable vitamin companies have now started to add herbs such as ginger to 'warm up' these formulae.
- Flax seed or linseed is also excellent as it not only delivers essential fatty acids but is a superb lubricant which can help to heal and repair inflamed tubes. You can buy raw linseeds (dark brown in colour) or a product called Linseed Gold, which is grown organically. You can also buy linseed oil (food grade quality, not to be confused with the oil used as a cricket bat sealer!). Ensure that these products are kept in a fridge to keep them from going rancid.
- Aloe vera juice cleanses, heals and soothes the bowel and is excellent for inflammatory bowel disorders. However, it is of a 'cool' nature, so cold individuals must ensure that their diet includes 'warming' foods to compensate.
- Slippery elm too has excellent healing properties as it coats the inner membranes of the digestive tract, thus allowing healing of the underlying tissues to take place.

Exercise

Too much lying down can damage the lung and large intestine meridians, affecting both elimination and respiration. To remedy this, work on acupressure point Large Intestine 4, located in the muscle between the thumb and first finger, and on Large Intestine 11, found at the elbow crease on the outer part of the arm (*see Figure, page 209*). While these points are being stimulated, make the lung sound 'SSSSS' and visualize the colour white healing and decongesting your large intestine.

An exercise to stretch the large intestine and lung meridians is described on page 188.

Deep breathing and relaxation exercises are very important to help re-educate the bowel. Remember that the lungs are the partner organ to the large intestine, so deep breathing will always have a positive impact on the bowels. See the exercises recommended on page 187.

Touch Therapies

Massage

Massaging the large intestine can be very therapeutic and helps to clear away some of the deposits that have built up over the years. Use an olive oil cream, or olive oil from the kitchen, to which a few drops of the essential oils recommended (*page 211*) have been added.

When undertaking any colon massage, it is important to drain the descending colon first, which is on the left-hand side.

1. Start by placing your hand just beneath your spleen on the left-hand side of your body. Using the heel of your hand, gently glide over the colon, feeling for any lumps and bumps. Passing the inside of the left hip bone, gently draw your hand towards your pubic bone. Repeat three times.
2. Move your hand to the liver region on the right-hand side, just beneath your ribs. Again, using the heel of your hand, gently glide it across to the left-hand side, noting any bumpy

patches, and down the descending colon as described in Step 1. Repeat three times.

3. Now move to the lowest point of the ascending colon, on the inside right hip. Glide the heel of your hand up towards the liver, three times.

4. Going back to the lowest point of the ascending colon, slide your hand up towards the liver area, across to the spleen, down the left hip and gently across to the pubic bone. Repeat three times.

5. Use your fingers to massage the whole colon area in a circular motion, following the (clockwise) direction of the colon, for a further two times. At this stage you can pay a little more attention to the knotted areas of the colon by massaging in small circles directly over them, moving on when they feel a little looser. This will begin to move the energy in the intestine and help relieve constipation.

Remember that your colon may have taken many years to get into its current state, so don't expect it to be clear after just a few sessions! You may notice that your bowel motions appear darker than usual. This just means that the old wastes that have built up and stuck to the walls of your intestine have been loosened and released. (However, if you see blood in your stool, consult your GP.)

There is also an extra area that is excellent to massage, if somewhat painful! The *fascia lata* muscle is located on the outside of the thigh from the knee to the top of the thigh, where the side seam of trousers would run. This muscle relates to the large intestine according to a therapy called Applied Kinesiology or Touch for Health. It will probably feel both tender and lumpy to the touch, but gently massaging this area with oil, or even just rubbing it through your trousers when you have a spare moment, will help to support the function of the large intestine.

Skin Brushing

Skin brushing is an excellent way to help detoxify the body, as the gentle friction on the skin stimulates the lymphatic system. In fact it is one of the best lymphatic cleansers known. When practised daily for a few months it can also improve body tone.

This treatment should be carried out on dry skin for about 3 minutes prior to having a shower or bath.

1. Starting from the feet, brush the soles as well as the upper side using a long-handled natural brush. Using long, sweeping strokes, brush up the legs, covering all of the skin's surface area, concentrating on the thighs and buttocks.
2. Put one arm up in the air, allowing gravity to help drain the lymph to the armpit, and sweep down the arm with gentle strokes, drawing towards the armpit.
3. Brush the torso by brushing towards the heart, and when doing the lower abdomen, brush up the right-hand side, just on the inside of the hip bone, across the transverse colon beneath the ribs and down the left-hand side, then gently across the pelvic area to complete the circle. Repeat.
4. When working near the breast area, brush over the top of the breast, always aiming for the armpit – and remember, be gentle over sensitive areas!

Your skin will become more resilient and you will be able to take more vigorous brushing after a few weeks. Visualize while you do this that your body is being cleansed and purified, with all the toxins being dredged into the lymphatic system to be released in the colon. Stools may contain large amounts of mucus after beginning skin brushing, which is a good sign that the body is beginning to clear away old matter. Skin brushing is subject to 'homeostatic resistance', in other words the body quite simply gets used to it. To over-ride this, it is best to follow a regular daily programme of skin brushing one to two times a day for three months, then reduce this to twice a week – preferably keeping to a regular routine.

The *pièce de résistance* is to take a warm shower and follow this with a quick blast of cold water. Apart from being highly stimulating, this encourages the dilation and contraction of the blood vessels and further incites movement of the lymph. You will also feel very invigorated – try it!

Reflexology

The colon is one of the more complicated reflexology zones to massage as you must start on the left foot and work on the ileo-caecal valve and ascending colon, across half of the transverse colon, and continue on to the right foot, still following the transverse colon until you move on to the descending colon and rectum. One easy-to-follow method is to massage this reflex in tiny circular movements (noting particularly 'gritty' areas), gradually working along the length of the colon. When you have completed this, you can return to the trouble spots and gently massage these again. (*See page 30 for massage techniques.*)

Reflexology points for the large intestine (shaded)

The large intestine meridian

Acupressure

The large intestine meridian begins at the outside tip of the index finger and travels to Large Intestine 4, a major point located in the webbing between the thumb and the index finger. It runs along the forearm and up to the shoulder and, after dividing into two channels, finishes at the nose.

This is a key point on the large intestine meridian, but should not be used on pregnant women. It is a valuable point that can help to detoxify the body by relieving constipation and improving the function of the large intestine. It is a good point to help improve the complexion. It can also relieve frontal headaches, shoulder pain and toothache. Good to massage when you are watching television!

Large Intestine 4 and 11 acupressure points

LARGE INTESTINE 11

To find this point, bend your elbow and take your thumb along the crease until you feel a slight depression before the bone. It will probably be tender! This is an effective point to massage to relieve constipation and stimulate a sluggish bowel. It is also a good point to foster a blooming complexion, especially if used in conjunction with LI 4.

Essential Oils

Fennel: rebalances the digestive system and stimulates the flow of energy in the large intestine, so helping with bloating and flatulence. Its antispasmodic properties can release tension held in the intestines. Encourages us to communicate and show our feelings rather than allowing them to fester. *Strength factor: Strong*

German chamomile: heals inflammation in the bowel, making it useful for diarrhoea and general bowel symptoms such as irritable bowel disease. If the cause of diarrhoea is an allergy to a certain food, this oil would be a good choice due to its calming, soothing and antispasmodic properties. *Strength factor: Strong*

If your stools are loose and you frequently suffer from diarrhoea, it is important to consider the possible causes. It could be too much cold food, nerves, allergies or parasites. If it has been triggered by a virus or bacterial infection, then Eucalyptus and Tea Tree oils would be most helpful. However, for stress-induced bowel problems brought on by excessive workloads, exams or an interview, for example, anti-spasmodic oils such as Lavender and Neroli can be used. The latter is especially good as a preventative to help alleviate stress and anxiety before they lead to diarrhoea. If there is much pain and cramp due to spasm of the intestinal muscles, try oil of Ginger combined with Fennel, as both are warming and carminative oils. Oil of Rosemary is an excellent bowel stimulant.

Emotions

The phrase 'to have the guts' to do something reflects the age-old belief that the large intestine holds sway over our courage and fortitude. When the large intestine is weak, we may not be able to fight the difficulties that face us and may lack determination, which can lead to disappointment, despair and bitterness. Just as the large intestine is continually working on waste in the body and chewing things over, the mind does the same thing psychologically. Petty behaviour, hanging on to negativity and continual dissatisfaction are some of the behaviour patterns to expect. We may become unable to appreciate anything or anyone, so can lose our family and friends and become isolated and lonely.

Grief is the emotion connected to the Metal element; it is well known that intense grief can have a profound impact on our health and well-being. If we have lost someone it is perfectly natural to grieve, but there does come a time when it is essential to 'let go'. Counselling and affirmations (*see page 214*) can greatly assist in this process. Do not forget deep breathing exercises, as these will not only remove stagnant carbon dioxide but will also move blood and oxygen into the lungs – the partner of the large intestine – to release congestion. While doing deep breathing exercises, be willing to repeat affirmations about letting go of the past, and visualize any grief and pain being 'let go' by your body.

People who cannot 'let go' retain all types of unnecessary garbage as problems are kept inside – as with constipation the body holds on to old rubbish that is no longer needed. Events that have happened in our past affect our behaviour and happiness in the present. Some people like to hang on to the past and blame others for their present unhappiness, instead of taking positive, decisive action to improve matters by learning to forgive. It is the ability to forgive that is important. If we cannot forgive ourselves, this can lead to self-destructive behaviour. All we can do is learn from our experiences – to become better, kinder and more positive human beings. We need to focus on positive, uplifting, nurturing thoughts and feelings and give less power to those negative, destructive thought patterns that only serve to reduce our energy levels and destroy joy and peace of mind. Try using the 'Law of Substitution': whenever a negative message begins to play in your head, stop it in its tracks and replace it with a positive affirmation. If you are too upset and cannot even focus on an affirmation, quietly say a simple word such as 'peace' and feel calmness filling your body and soul.

Flower Remedies

Crab Apple: known as the cleansing remedy. For those wishing to purify the body. Indicated when there are feelings of being 'unclean': Dr Bach described it as '*the remedy which helps us to get rid of anything we do not like either in our minds or bodies*'. Helps us to process negativity, impurities and unresolved issues.

Honeysuckle: for when your life has got 'stuck in the past'. For those who romanticize over past times and are nostalgic, often missing the present times as they are so preoccupied with dwelling on the past. Focuses the mind on the here and now so we can learn to put the past into its proper perspective.

Pine: for those who carry feelings of guilt, often when the wrongdoing is not of their own making. Initiates the process of forgiveness and invokes feelings of genuine regret rather than guilt.

Walnut: known as the 'link breaker', helping to break negative thought patterns and encouraging us to let go, move on and cultivate more positive and nourishing thoughts. Dr Bach called it *'the remedy for those who have decided to take a great step forward in life, to break old conventions, to leave old limits and restrictions and start on a new way'*.

You may also find some appropriate flower remedies for supporting the Metal element in the chapter on the lungs (page 196).

Affirmations

- I trust my large intestine to eliminate all waste products from my body easily.
- I now forgive myself and others, so enabling me to move forward in life.
- My skin covers and protects my whole body and is healthy, clear and glowing.
- It is safe for me to process and release anything that is no longer needed by my mind, body and spirit.

See also the lungs chapter, page 196, for affirmations that may be used in conjunction with these.

Meditation for the Metal Element
See lungs chapter, page 196.

Creating a Naturally Better Future

Despite the differences between conventional and natural medicine, both Eastern and Western approaches have their value for the sick patient. So often we take for granted that Western methods are the best, but the ancient wisdom of the East can make an equally important contribution; perhaps an optimal approach to future healthcare may be a combined approach. Natural medicine and traditional healing methods are undoubtedly excellent long-term approaches to maintaining health, as they are gentle yet highly effective. However, conventional medicine is appropriate in certain situations including life-threatening emergencies and those that require surgery. Eastern and Western methods should become more integrated in the next decade as we move towards a truly eclectic medical system where the chief objective should be to restore balance, harmonious function and wellbeing.

The notion of healing yourself is at the root of the natural and Chinese medicine philosophy. As more individuals have witnessed first-hand the harmful effects that occur due to the over-use or misuse of modern medical drugs, they are turning to gentler, less invasive techniques that do not have such a disruptive effect on the body and which invoke self-healing. We need to recognize that the individual can play a fundamental role in his or her own healing process.

In today's society, we have forgotten how to create the right conditions for the body to heal itself. Factors such as inappropriate lifestyle, poor diet and the polluted environment we have created, all abuse the delicate working systems of our body. For millions of years, man has been eating a simple diet of unrefined, organic produce, yet in this century we have resorted to using technology and chemicals to process, and consequently adulterate, our food. I believe it is now time for us all to take responsibility for our precious Mother Earth who sustains, nurtures and supports us with food, water and healing plants. We should never take her gifts for granted; we should respect her and give thanks for all that she supplies. We should nurture her in the same way that we should nurture ourselves.

The wisdom lies within.

Further Reading and Resources

The Natural Medicines Society
Market Chambers
13a Market Place
Heanor
Derbyshire DE75 7AA
Tel: 01773 710002

British Complementary Medicine Association
35 Prestbury Road
Cheltenham
Glos GS5Q 2PT
Tel: 01242 226770

British Holistic Medical Association
Trust House
Royal Shrewsbury Hospital South
Shrewsbury SY3 8XF
Tel: 01743 261155

Institute for Complementary Medicine
PO Box 194
London SE16 1QZ
Tel: 0171 237 5165
(Please send a SAE with two first class stamps.)

Aromatherapy

Davis, Patricia. *Aromatherapy: an A–Z*, C. W. Daniel, 1995
Hopkins, Cathy. *Principles of Aromatherapy*, Thorsons, 1996
Lawless, Julia. *The Encyclopaedia of Essential Oils*, Element Books, 1992
Mojay, Gabriel. *Aromatherapy for Healing the Spirit*, Gaia Books, 1996
Price, Shirley. *Practical Aromatherapy*, Thorsons, 1994
— *Shirley Price's Aromatherapy Workbook: understanding essential oils*,
Thorsons, 1993
Sellar, Wanda. *The Directory of Essential Oils*, C. W. Daniel, 1992
Worwood, Valerie Ann. *The Fragrant Pharmacy: a complete guide to
aromatherapy and essential oils*, Bantam Books, 1991

The Aromatherapy Organisations Council
3 Latymer Close
Braybrooke
Market Harborough
Leics LE16 8LN
Tel: 01858 434242

International Federation of Aromatherapists
Stamford House
2–4 Chiswick High Road
London W4 1TH
Tel: 0181 742 2605

The International Society of Professional Aromatherapists
82 Ashby Road
Hinkley
Leics LE10 1SN
Tel: 01455 637987

Fleur Organic Essential Oils
Pembroke Studios
Pembroke Road
London N10 2JE
Tel: 0181 444 1424   Fax: 0181 444 0704

Neal's Yard
15 Neal's Yard
Covent Garden
London WC2H 9FP
Mail order: 0161 831 7875

Tisserand Aromatherapy Products Ltd
Newtown Road
Hove
Sussex BN3 7BA
Tel: 01273 325666   Fax: 01273 208444

Chinese Medicine

Chia, Mantak and Maneewan. *Chi Nei Tsang: internal organs chi - massage*, Healing Tao Books, 1991

Connelly, Dianne M. *Traditional Acupuncture: the law of the five elements*, Traditional Acupuncture Institute, 1994

Firebrace, Peter and Hill, Sandra. *A Guide to Acupuncture*, Constable, 1994

Hicks, Angela. *Principles of Chinese Medicine*, Thorsons, 1996

Kaptchuk, Ted J. *Chinese Medicine: the web has no weaver*, Century Paperbacks, 1987

Maciocia, Giovanni. *The Foundations of Chinese Medicine*, Churchill Livingstone, 1989

Dr Mann, Felix. *Textbook of Acupuncture*, Butterworth-Heinemann, 1993

Teeguarden, Iona Marsaa. *Acupressure Way of Health: Jin Shin Do*, Japan Publications, 1978

Page, Michael. *The Power of Ch'i: introduction to Chinese mysticism and philosophy*, Aquarian Press, 1994

Gach, Michael Reed. *Acupressure: how to cure common ailments the natural way*, Piatkus Books, 1993

Soo, Hilda. *The Chinese Art of T'ai Chi Ch'uan*, Aquarian Press, 1984

Tierra, Lesley. *Herbs of Life: health and healing using Western and Chinese techniques*, USA, Crossing Press, 1992

Williams, Tom PhD. *Chinese Medicine: Acupuncture, Herbal Remedies, Nutrition, Qigong and Health Essentials*, Element Books, 1995

Young, Jacqueline. *Acupressure for Health: a complete self-care manual*, Thorsons, 1994

British Acupuncture Council
206–208 Latimer Road
London W10 6RE
Tel: 0181 964 0222

Flower Remedies

Harvey, Clare G. and Cochrane, Amanda. *The Encyclopaedia of Flower Remedies: a guide to the healing power of,* Thorsons, 1995
Scheffer, Mechthild. *Bach Flower Therapy: theory and practice,* Thorsons, 1986
The Work of Dr Edward Bach, Wigmore Publications, 1995

Dr Edward Bach Foundation
Mount Vernon
Sotwell
Wallingford OX10 0PZ
Customer services: 0181 780 4200

Healing Herbs' Bach Flower Remedies
PO Box 65
Hereford HR2 0UW
Tel: 01873 890218

The Nutri-Centre
The Hale Clinic
7 Park Crescent
London W1N 3HE
Tel: 0171 436 5122
(Sells Bach remedies, Jan de Vries Essences, Planetary Formulas, Blue-Green Algae, nutritional supplements e.g. Biocare, Solgar.)

Herbalism

Tierra, Lesley. *The Herbs of Life: health and healing using Western and Chinese techniques,* USA, Crossing Press, 1992

Tierra, Michael. *Planetary Herbology*, USA, Lotus Light Publications, 1989
— *The Natural Remedy Bible*, Pocket Books, 1994
Mills, Simon. *The Complete Guide to Modern Herbalism*, Thorsons, 1994
Hoffman, David. *Thorsons Guide to Medical Herbalism*, Thorsons, 1991
de Vries, Jan. By Appointment Only series, e.g. *Traditional Home and Herbal Remedies* (1986), *How to Live a Healthy Life* (1995), *Questions and Answers on Family Health* (1994), Mainstream Publishing Company
Dr Vogel, H. C. A. *Nature Doctor: manual of traditional medicine*, Mainstream Publishing Company, 1990

East West College of Herbalism
Hartswood
Marsh Green
Hartfield
East Sussex TN7 4ET
Tel: 01342 822312

Register of Chinese Herbal Medicine
PO Box 400
Wembley
Middlesex HA9 9NZ
Tel: 0181 904 1357

National Institute of Medical Herbalists
56 Longbrook Street
Exeter EX4 6AH
Tel: 01392 426022

Homoeopathy

The Society of Homoeopaths
2 Artizan Road
Northampton NN1 4HU
Tel: 01604 21400

United Kingdom Homoeopathic Medical Association
6 Livingstone Road
Gravesend
Kent DA12 5DZ
Tel: 01474 560336

Nutrition and Healing

Chaitow, Leon. *Holistic Pain Relief*, Thorsons, 1996

—, *Candida Albicans*, Thorsons, 1996

Dr Davies, Stephen and Dr Stewart, Alan. *Nutritional Medicine: the drug-free guide to better family health*, Pan Books, 1987

Grant, Doris and Joice, Jean. *Food Combining for Health*, Thorsons, 1991

Haas, Elson M. MD. *Staying Healthy with Nutrition*, Celestial Arts, 1992

Kenton, Leslie. *Lean Revolution*, Ebury Press, 1994

—, *10 Day De-Stress Plan*, Ebury Press, 1994

—, *10 Steps to Energy*, Ebury Press, 1997

Hay, Louise L. *Heal Your Body: the mental causes for physical illness*, Eden Grove Editions, 1989

Lazarides, Linda. *Principles of Nutritional Therapy*, Thorsons, 1996

Lidolt, Erwina. *The Food Combining Cookbook: recipes for the Hay system*, 1987

Lu, Henry C. *Chinese System of Food Cures: prevention and remedies*, USA, Sterling Publications, 1986

Marsden, Kathryn. *The Food Combining Diet: lose weight and stay healthy with the Hay system*, Thorsons, 1993

Dr Northrup, Christiane. *Women's Bodies, Women's Wisdom: the complete guide to women's health*, Piatkus, 1995

Dr Page, Christine. *Frontiers of Health: from healing to wholeness*, C. W. Daniel, 1992

—, *The Mirror of Existence: stepping into wholeness*, C. W. Daniel, 1995

Smyth, Angela, edited by Dr Jones, Hilary. *The Complete Encyclopaedia of Natural Health*, Thorsons, 1997

Dr Werbach, Melvyn. *Healing through Nutrition: the natural approach to treating illnesses*, Thorsons, 1995

British Association for Counselling
1 Regent Place
Rugby CV21 2PJ
Tel: 01788 578328

National Federation of Spiritual Healers
Old Manor Farm Studio
Church Street
Sunbury-on-Thames
Middlesex TW6 6RG
Tel: 01932 783164   Healer referral line: 0891 616080

General Council and Register of Naturopaths
Goswell House
Goswell Road
Street
Somerset BA16 0JG
Tel: 01458 840072

Society for the Promotion of Nutritional Therapy
PO Box 47
Heathfield
East Sussex TN21 8ZX
Tel: 01435 867007

Register of Nutritional Therapists
Hatton Green
Warwick CV35 7LA

Jennifer Harper
PO Box 150
Woking
Surrey GU23 6XS

Reflexology

Bayly, Doreen E. *Reflexology Today: the stimulation of the body's healing forces through foot massage*, Healing Arts Press, 1982
Kunz, Kevin and Barbara. *The Complete Guide to Foot Reflexology*, Thorsons, 1984
—, *Hand and Food Reflexology*, Thorsons, 1986

Association of Reflexologists
27 Old Gloucester Street
London WC1N 3XX
Tel: 01990 673320

Organic Produce

The Soil Association
86 Colston Street
Bristol BS1 5BB
Tel: 0117 929 0661

Choice Organics
Unit 2, Bridges Wharf
Bridges Court
off York Road
London SW11 3QS
Tel: 0171 924 1744   Fax: 0171 924 1330
(Delivers organic food and eco-friendly products.)

Pipers Farm (meat)
Peter and Henrietta Greig
Pipers Farm
Cullompton
Devon EX15 1SD
Tel: 01392 881380   Fax: 01392 881600